FIGHTING DISEASE

THE COMPLETE GUIDE TO

NATURAL IMMUNE POWER

BY ELLEN MICHAUD, ALICE FEINSTEIN
AND THE EDITORS OF *PREVENTION* MAGAZINE

MEDICAL ADVISER: TERRY PHILLIPS, PH.D.
Director of the Immunogenetics and Immunochemistry Laboratories
George Washington University Medical Center, Washington, D.C.

 Rodale Press, Emmaus, Pennsylvania

Prevention magazine is a registered trademark of Rodale Press, Inc.

Printed in the United States of America on acid-free paper ∞

Book design by Acey Lee
Illustrations by Greg Imhoff

If you have any questions or comments concerning this book, please write:
    Rodale Press
    Book Reader Service
    33 East Minor Street
    Emmaus, PA 18098

Library of Congress Cataloging-in-Publication Data

Michaud, Ellen.
    Fighting disease : the complete guide to natural immune power / by Ellen Michaud,
  Alice Feinstein, and the editors of Prevention magazine ; medical adviser, Terry Phillips.
        p.   cm.
    Includes index.
    ISBN 0-87857-830-7   hardcover
    1. Natural immunity – Popular works.   2. Health.   I. Feinstein, Alice.   II. Phillips,
  Terry M.   III. Prevention (Emmaus, Pa.)   IV. Title.
  QR185.2.M53   1989
  616.07'9 – dc20   89-6223
                                                                                                        CIP

Distributed in the book trade by St. Martin's Press

2 4 6 8 10 9 7 5 3   hardcover

Contributors

Editors: Carol Keough, John Feltman

Contributing Writers: William LeGro, Lance Jacobs

Editorial/Production Coordinator: Jane Sherman

Copy Editor: Lisa D. Andruscavage

Research Coordinator: Karen Lombardi

Research Staff: **Ann Gossy, Susan A. Nastasee, Holly Clemson,** Christine Dreisbach, Karen Feridun, Staci Hadeed, Dawn Horvath, Bernadette Sukley

Office Staff: **Roberta Mulliner,** Stacy Brobst, Lori Engelman, Deborah Maher, Kelly Trumbauer

Vice President and Editor in Chief, Prevention Magazine Health Books: William Gottlieb

Group Vice President, Health: Mark Bricklin

CONTENTS

ACKNOWLEDGMENTS

The human immune system presents a complex and beautiful panorama that is only beginning to yield its secrets to humanity. We'd like to thank all those who journeyed with us on our path to translating these exciting new discoveries into practical healing information. We'd like to especially thank all the physicians and researchers we interviewed, who took time from their vital work to share their findings with the general public; our editor, Carol Keough, who has (and needed) the patience of a saint; our medical adviser, Terry Phillips, Ph.D., whose attention to nuance and detail helped keep us on the straight and narrow; contributing writer William LeGro, whose endless hours of interviews and thought contributed so much to this book; librarian Janet Glassman, whose personal dedication and computer expertise allowed us to send our curiosity searching through the thousands of theories, thoughts, and studies buried in scientific journals from around the world; our research coordinator, Karen Lombardi, who left no sentence unturned in the quest for accuracy; and our families, who are by now immune to our rantings about microbes, phagocytes, and vaccinations.

INTRODUCTION: WHAT THIS BOOK CAN DO FOR YOU

Suddenly, you have an immune system.

Your immune system existed long before the advent of AIDS, but you probably didn't pay much attention to it. If you are like most people, you barely knew it existed.

Of course, it's been there all along. From the day you were born, billions of specialized immune cells in your body went silently about their business of protecting you from disease. Spectacular cell wars raged within you every day as invading microbes were captured and destroyed. But the drama played to an empty house. Except for a few specialists laboring anonymously in their laboratories, no one paid much attention to the vital functions of the immune system. No one talked about it. Until recently.

Then came AIDS. It was as if the lights were switched on, the volume went up, and the curtain rose. There was this new star out on center stage: your immune system. And the public didn't know when to applaud because they didn't understand the performance. What exactly *is* the immune system? What exactly does it do and how does it work? And most important, what can we do to help it do its job better? Is there any way to coax it from the sidelines? Keep it healthy? Encourage a better performance?

Step right this way. Here's your program.

This book introduces you to a vital, vibrant part of yourself. Read chapter 2, The Inner Workings, to find out how your immune system saves your life every day. This chapter acquaints you with the various components of your disease-fighting cellular army and provides a blow-by-blow description of its defensive strategy. You review the troops. You watch them in action. You may be surprised at the violence that exists within you, but when you realize that your health is the prize in this war against disease, you will want to know everything that you can do to help your immune system win.

Of course, if you want to get right into the practical advice, feel free to turn to part 2, An Immune Power Encyclopedia. It can be used as a ready reference for quick information about different aspects of the immune system. Or it can be read straight through for an overall look at the latest discoveries in how to help your immune system achieve peak performance.

As you are gleaning helpful hints from the various entries in this section, you may from time to time run across a term that you don't know. If you do, look it up in chapter 3, The Cast of Characters. This quick and easy reference section serves as a kind of dictionary of the immune system. Written in easy-to-understand language, this chapter helps you keep track of the key players.

In An Immune Power Encyclopedia, you'll find out about what foods your immune system needs to function at its optimum power. You'll find new inspiration to quit smoking, exercise, and get a good night's sleep. You'll discover that stress and negative emotions like grief really do make you more susceptible to illness. And you'll find out what you can do to short-circuit the devastating impact of such killer emotions.

Part 2 is also chock-full of helpful hints about how to assist your immune system in its battles with disease-causing microbes – how to germproof your kitchen, what shots you need as an adult, when and how to take antibiotics, how to prevent yeast infections, even how to treat a cut or burn. You'll find out that you no longer have to suffer from your allergies, why you must protect yourself from overexposure to the sun or from exposure to certain pesticides, and why you can't afford to ignore a sore throat.

In addition to hints about what you can do *now* to help your immune system, An Immune Power Encyclopedia takes a look at researchers' latest insights into some of humanity's worst scourges – cancer, arthritis, Alzheimer's disease. Researchers hold out hope that through manipulating the immune system, some of these diseases may someday yield their ground.

And if you *really* want to get into bringing your immune system up to its optimum fighting power, turn to part 3, How to Build a Strong Immune System. This section provides you with a day-to-day agenda for strengthening your immune system. The program will help you put together lifestyle changes – everything from diet to stress-busters – that will help you boost your immune functioning up to where it should be. Think of Your 30-Day Immune Power Program as basic training for the cellular troops. When you finish implementing this program, you should have an immune fighting army at your service that's ready to meet its daily challenges.

Part I
How Your Immune System Works

1

THE INNER WORKINGS: SELF-PRESERVATION

Outwardly you may be a gentle, peaceful person, a loving parent, a churchgoer, even a pacifist. Inside of you, however, whether you will it or not, an awesome fighting force is on alert. The human immune system is an efficient war machine that never negotiates a treaty. It strikes no bargains with the enemy. It takes no prisoners.

Microbes that dare contemplate taking up residence inside your nice warm body encounter a standing army of trained warrior cells, willing to martyr themselves in defense of the cause – your health and well-being. Enemies are exploded, dissolved, digested to death, and carried out of your body until the very last enemy is eliminated. Peace finally returns to your sinews and tissues, but even then your immune system is not finished. It prepares a dossier on the enemy so that if any more of them show up, they will be recognized and dispatched even more quickly the next time. That's how you became immune to diseases like mumps or chickenpox.

In the microscopic world, the rule is kill or be killed. If your immune system didn't fight for you every day of your life, you would not be alive to read this page. It is one army that can't afford to relax its discipline.

The human immune system is a fighting force of intricate beauty, exquisite in its potent complexity, and alas, very necessary. If you have the courage to face the more violent side of your own nature, let's review the troops.

MEET THE ENEMY

Before you can really appreciate the warrior cells inside you and their lethal arsenal, consider the enemy. Bacteria, viruses, an assortment of yeasts, fungi, and parasites – they don't look like much. You can't even

1

see them without the aid of a microscope, but they have you surrounded. Just outside the all-too-penetrable borders of your body, just outside your skin and mucous membranes, swarms a horde of countless tiny creatures that would like nothing better than to turn your body into a microbe housing project.

You are warm. Your blood and tissues are engorged with a continual supply of water and life-giving nutrients. You want to keep this space inside you just for you, but this multitude of microbes views your body as a good place to raise a family. When they do successfully cross the border, breach your lines of defense, and entrench themselves inside of you, their collective presence is called an infection.

You think it's okay to share? Think maybe there's enough food and shelter inside you for both your own cells and assorted microbial families? Think again. These infections have names like tuberculosis, leprosy, malaria, the common cold, plague, influenza – all the ills to which the human species is heir.

And there are so many microbes to contend with. More than a million bacteria swarm on every square inch of your *freshly washed* skin. You carry them to your mouth with every forkful of food. You inhale them in the very air you breathe.

Something as seemingly harmless as a coworker's sneeze translates into warfare for your immune system. A sneeze reportedly explodes from the mouth and nostrils at 40 miles per hour, as opposed to the relatively gentle 5 miles per hour for normal breathing. And hitching a ride on every minute droplet expelled by that sneeze are countless homeless viruses, all hoping to encounter someone just like *you.* You take one breath of this virus-laden air, and your immune system has to call in the reserves.

IMMUNE ARMY MARCHES

What actually happens when your immune defenses turn on is startlingly complex. Immune system lectures are considered among the most difficult in medical school, says Edwin Cooper, Ph.D., professor of anatomy and cell biology at UCLA School of Medicine.

"All of these immune cells we're talking about have to be born someplace. That place is in the bone marrow. The bone marrow is just a great big nursery ward with little 'babies' in it, and it's hard to tell which one is which. Medical students just pull their hair," says Dr. Cooper.

Every day, your bone marrow nursery pours out millions of new red and white blood cells. The red cells carry oxygen for you and the white cells constitute your standing army against disease. Let's meet the different types of white blood cells, and let's meet them out on the battlefield. They are a lot easier to understand when you watch them in action.

Let's watch what happens during a localized infection. For this little exercise, we'll need a splinter. You've just hauled some kindling in for the fireplace, and if you'll check that red spot there on your palm, you'll find just what we need. Now just shrink down to microscopic size for a moment and let's take a closer look.

The opening scene in this little drama is deceptively peaceful. A number of bacteria rode in on that splinter, and they think they've died and gone to microbe heaven. They are already cavorting about in the spaces between your muscle cells and slurping up food. These uninvited immigrants have found so much liquid nourishment there for the taking that they are already multiplying. There are more and more and more of them. Bacteria multiply exponentially. That means that 2 become 4, 4 become 8, 8 become 16, and so on. It doesn't take a particularly good mathematician to realize that all these little creatures secreting their toxins can soon become a very big problem for their host – *if* they are allowed to carry on their dining and reproductive activities unmolested, that is.

Unbeknownst to this unsavory multitude of microbes, their doom is already sealed. When that splinter broke the skin, a silent chemical alarm went off. The blood in the immediate area started getting "sticky." Blood cells started hanging up on the capillary vessel walls and slowing down. Blood cells keep arriving, however, making the area slightly swollen and tender. The increased blood flow and tenderness in the area is known as the inflammatory response.

In a few moments, white blood cells start to crawl right *through* the capillary walls. They actually leave the blood vessels and head right for the splinter. Now the bacteria are really in for it. There are several different kinds of white blood cells that are likely to get involved in the ensuing battle.

SHOCK TROOPS ARRIVE

First on the scene are the neutrophils. The shock troops of the immune system, these cells are numerous, constituting 60 to 75 percent of your white blood cells.

"They are the ones that get really excited when an infection comes. When you get a splinter in your finger, they are the ones that rush there like mad and gather around the splinter and just 'chew' away at it," says

Dr. Cooper. "Some of them die in the process. That's how you get pus. Pus is a mass of dead neutrophils that have just engorged themselves to death. They go there and clean up the mess and some of them die there and *they* get cleaned up until the whole wound is taken care of."

Dr. Cooper uses the word "chew" advisedly. He knows neutrophils don't have any teeth. Actually, they don't have a mouth either. So, you might ask, how do they manage to consume all those invading bacteria?

Did you ever see an amoeba? If you saw one through a microscope in high school you probably remember it. If not, picture some clear jelly in a glass of water. Now imagine that the jelly is animated and can kind of flow around at will. When it wants to go in a particular direction, it oozes out a part of itself (that would be a pseudopod), and then the rest of it just catches up by flowing into the extended pseudopod.

A neutrophil is just like an amoeba except that instead of being an independent creature, it lives inside you and in fact forms a part of your blood. It moves by sliding here and there. And it eats by enveloping its meal with its body.

Take an unsuspecting bacterium. Put an aggressive neutrophil next to it, and the neutrophil will ooze on over and engulf it. The bacterium experiences death by digestion.

TANK CORPS ROLLS IN

Behind the neutrophil, another amoebalike cell crawls up to get into the action. Behold the macrophage. Though fewer in number and slower than neutrophils, the macrophage is a whole lot bigger. In fact, *macro* means "big" and *phage* means "eater." This big, cell-eating monster views all those bacteria as so many orders of hamburgers and french fries. It eats and it goes back for seconds, and then it eats some more.

It seems the more the macrophage eats, the more it gets turned on to the job. Macrophages tend to hang around in your tissues minding their own business. When a chemical signal brings the heat of nearby battle to their attention, they move in like some primeval tank corps called into action. Once they arrive on the scene, they liven up. They move faster, seemingly delighted with the microbial banquet.

Macrophages also do burial detail. The battle scene can get quite messy, with dead neutrophils and exploded bits of cellular debris piling up fast. Macrophages are indiscriminate eaters. They digest the pus and eventually leave a wound antiseptically clean. In fact, some macrophages live a life devoted solely to clean-up duties. They line your lungs and carry off stray bits of dust, pollens, and pollutants that sneak past the filtering system in your nostrils. If you happen to be a smoker, they turn black in their efforts to eat up all the tar and carbon deposits that reach your lungs.

Macrophages have one spectacular talent that distinguishes them from neutrophils, but before we get to that, we need to meet one more white blood cell.

TURN OFF TURNCOATS

All the immune cells we've met so far are *nonspecific,* meaning that they'll go after anything that isn't you. The natural killer cell, alias the NK cell, is also considered to be a somewhat nonspecific cell, but it goes after things that *are* you. Sort of.

Every army in the world deals harshly with traitors. Just one successful Benedict Arnold can undermine a country's defenses. Similarly, one cancer cell that goes undetected can grow into a life-threatening tumor. Natural killer cells conduct constant surveillance, looking for cells that have gone bad – tumor cells that could kill you if allowed to grow unchallenged.

A tumor cell is a body cell that is out of whack. It has begun to multiply unnaturally and is not behaving at all like it should. When the natural killer cell makes its rounds and happens upon certain types of tumor cells, it carries out an execution.

"There's got to be contact. If you do some electron microscopy, using powerful optics to look at the immune system the same way we view stars through a telescope, you can see the intimate contact between the target cell and the killer cell," says Dr. Cooper. "Scientists assume there's something like a killer substance that's passed from the killer cell to the target that zaps it and kills it. Killer cells have these granules of enzymes or poisons. When the contact occurs, these granules will move down toward the area of intimate contact and sort of sit there. It's assumed the killer cell is passing weapons across the cell membrane to kill the tumor cell. NK cells do multiple killing. They can latch onto one cell, kill it, detach, pass around, and find another one and zap that one, too. They're pretty efficient."

GET SPECIFIC

So far, all the warrior cells that we've met can take on multiple opponents. They're specialized killers, tough little fighters that live only to die for you.

But the macrophage, remember, has one additional talent. After it finishes its meal, it burps out pieces of the enemy and puts them out on its surface to show them to an entirely separate class of immune cells known as lymphocytes. It's as though the macrophage is preparing an appetizer tray to entice these lymphocytes to get into the action. Once the lymphocytes decide to march into battle, your immune system has launched a full-power counterattack.

The lymphocytes are white blood cells that have been educated to attack *specific* targets. They are your killer elite, an elaborate network of cells that form what is known as your specific immune system. If the neutrophils and macrophages are the foot soldiers, then the various types of lymphocytes serve as the commissioned officers. There are two main categories of lymphocytes: T-cells and B-cells. Although they look very much alike under an ordinary microscope, they are distinguished by where they got their "educations" and by the kinds of weapons they carry into battle.

Both kinds of lymphocytes are born in the bone marrow. Those that are genetically programmed to become T-cells journey to the thymus, a two-lobed gland that sits in the upper portion of the chest at the base of the neck. When they later emerge from the thymus, they have somehow learned how to function as T-cells. Those that are programmed to be B-cells remain in the bone marrow to mature and learn their function. Once T-cells leave the thymus and B-cells leave the marrow, the cell types lodge in your lymph nodes, tonsils, spleen, and certain tissues in your gut.

Once they've completed their "educations," what distinguishes the two main categories of lymphocytes is their weapons systems, says Michael Lieber, M.D., Ph.D., immunologist with the National Institutes of Health. The B-cells hurl chemical spears, while the T-cells carry chemical swords, he says. That is, the T-cells have to bump right up against the enemy in order to dispatch it, while the B-cells do their killing from a distance.

Both B-cells and T-cells are programmed to respond to only a few enemies each. They have what might be described as chemical keys on their surfaces. The enemy microbes possess the equivalent of chemical locks. When a lymphocyte encounters an enemy that its key fits, fireworks happen – the immune system goes to war. You have millions of these lymphocytes within you, and collectively they form a protective net that successfully turns back every invasion. If your immune system *does* lose one of its wars, you'll be the first to know.

DIAL B FOR BLITZ

Let's watch what happens when B-cells are called into action. B-cells are fairly laid back. They tend to hang around in your spleen and lymph nodes, rather like bored recruits restricted to base.

On this particular afternoon a macrophage fresh from a gastrointestinal battle with salmonella wanders into a lymph node with bits of the bacteria clinging to its surface. It shows its trophies to one B-cell after another and gets no response. Finally, it contacts a B-cell that is programmed to recognize that particular type of bacteria. *Wow! How dare this dangerous creature show up here. Red alert! Red alert! Action!*

And, like Clark Kent stepping into a phone booth to come out as Superman, the B-cell undergoes a marvelous transformation that turns it into a plasma cell.

"It's a beautiful cell to look at once it becomes a plasma cell," says Dr. Cooper. "It's blue under the microscope. It's pear shaped. The nucleus fits down into the small part of the pear and the nuclear outline, or chromatin in the nucleus, has a very characteristic arrangement. We call it a clock-faced nucleus. This is the plasma cell, or stimulated B-lymphocyte. It then makes and pours out antibodies."

DIAL Y FOR GOOD-BYE

Antibodies, the chemical spears we mentioned earlier, are proteins shaped like the letter Y. The plasma cell secretes tailor-made antibodies on its surface that will fit exactly onto the enemy that stimulated it into action. If a salmonella bacterium turns on a B-cell, the stimulated B-cell will pour out antibodies designed to glom on to salmonella and thus inactivate it.

When antibodies, which move through the blood like homing missiles, encounter their target, they set off a chain reaction designed to blast holes in the enemy's membranes. First the two prongs of the Y stick onto the bacteria or whatever is being zapped. That leaves the pointy end of the Y hanging out there like yet another chemical key.

In this case, a complicated series of proteins known as complement have the right chemical keys to fit the antibodies' chemical locks. It takes components of complement plus antibodies to kill a bacterium. They all lock on together, and KA-BAM – good-bye salmonella.

One plasma cell vigorously pumping out antibodies does not a successful counterattack make. Bacteria reproduce too fast. No problem.

The plasma cell warrior has not yet played its full hand. It begins cloning itself, making multiple copies of itself. Soon there is a whole squadron of plasma cells firing antibody missiles at the distant salmonella invasion.

Antibodies also serve to call neutrophils and macrophages to the feast. While they might have missed an ungarnished bacterium, once the bacteria are slathered with antibodies, they are ever so much more appetizing.

DIAL T FOR TERMINATE

Viruses are special little creatures that present a particular challenge to your immune system. Bacteria take up residence between the cells of your body and do their damage through the toxins they secrete. Viruses are much smaller than bacteria. As one researcher described it, if you think of *E. coli* (a type of bacteria commonly found in your gut) as a football field, then a polio virus would be the size of the football.

Viruses are tricky. Shaped like minuscule jewels or tiny rocket ships, they are only partly alive. They can't reproduce without your help. In order to produce offspring, they need to slip *inside* the very cells of your body and snatch the DNA, the genetic stuff of life that you have bound up inside the nucleus of every cell.

Once inside the nucleus of one of your cells, viruses take over and turn the DNA into a little factory that manufactures more viruses. When the cell finally dies, thousands of new viruses can spew out, all looking to snatch other body cells to turn into new virus factories.

Macrophages and neutrophils can't do too much against a viral attack. This is a job for a specialist – the T-cell. Some researchers believe that T-cells may have evolved specifically to deal with viral invaders. T-cells, each one capable of spotting a different enemy, circulate through-out your body looking for just such intruders. You might think a virus would be well hidden inside a cell. Not so. In order to slip inside a cell, a virus has to remove its protein coat, which it leaves outside on the cell membrane.

The viral coat hanging outside signals the passing T-cell that viral hanky-panky is going on inside. Like the jealous husband who spots a strange jacket in the hall closet and *knows* what's going on in the upstairs bedroom, the T-cell takes swift action. It bumps against the body cell with the virus inside and perforates it. That quick destruction shuts down the virus assembly line.

The T-cell has no choice but to kill. It might be your own cell, but it's a goner, says Dr. Lieber. Like the creatures in the sci-fi movie *Invasion*

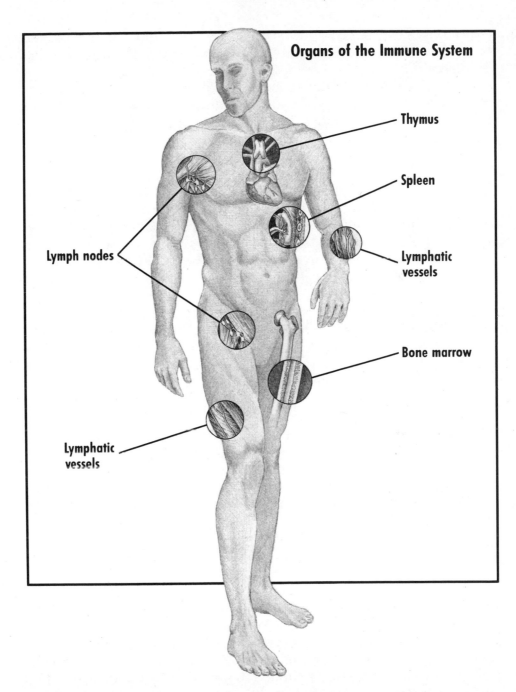

Organs of the Immune System

Thymus

Spleen

Lymph nodes

Lymphatic vessels

Bone marrow

Lymphatic vessels

The human immune system must protect every square inch of the body, both inside and out. In addition to specific organs, the immune system includes billions of warrior cells that patrol the entire body, on the lookout for any signs of trouble.

of the Body Snatchers, the viruses have snatched your cell. The immune system can't afford to show the cell any mercy because it is now working for the enemy.

A T-cell can kill only one sick cell at a time, however. What happens when one of those viral factories has already delivered up its first load of thousands of viruses? Once a T-cell is onto an invasion, it pulls off the same trick as the plasma cell. The T-cell clones itself. These duplicates, primed to respond to that particular enemy virus, also scurry about killing virus-infected cells.

Besides the killer T-cells (sometimes called effector T-cells) described here, there are also helper and suppressor T-cells. *Somebody* has to make strategic decisions. Helper T-cells check out the action and let the other components of the immune system know how big a defense to mount, how many antibodies are needed, how many clones to make. And suppressor T-cells watch the progress of the battle and call things to a halt when the final microbial corpse is carried from the field.

After any war, a few old soldiers live on to tell their tales, and so it is with the immune system. A few lymphocytes that remember what the enemy looks like continue to circulate in your blood just in case it shows up again. When you have some of these experienced old warrior cells on patrol for you, you are immune to the particular disease that they remember.

WHAT'S THE PASSWORD?

The immune system's cellular troops have your entire body under constant surveillance. Yet they don't have eyes with which to see. They don't have ears with which to hear. How can they tell an invading virus from a piece of your pancreas? How do they know a bacterium is not a brain cell?

They know because every single cell in your body is issued a badge of identification. The badge is actually a special arrangement of protein molecules as unique to you as your fingerprints. It says that you are you. Patrolling immune cells give everything that comes past them a little chemical feel. When a passing cell or pollen grain comes along and it's not wearing this badge of identification, its game is up.

Similarly, when one of your own cells goes bad and becomes a tumor cell, something on its surface is apparently not quite right. It is unclear just how a natural killer cell spots a tumor cell, but it seems there is some sort of a surface marker that betrays it.

Sometimes the immune system gets a little confused about who is wearing a badge and who isn't. It sometimes mistakes components of your own body for the enemy. When the immune system turns against the body, the result is called autoimmunity. This immune system confusion is behind a whole host of diseases, from rheumatoid arthritis to multiple sclerosis.

When things go right, as they usually do, your immune system keeps you healthy. If you don't like the idea of a military regime marching around inside you and making war without your conscious approval, you might take heart in the thought that your own internal army is purely defensive. It doesn't go out looking for trouble. It responds only when attacked. The violence of your immune system keeps you alive to think your thoughts of peace.

2

THE CAST
OF CHARACTERS

Now that you've seen how your immune system works, let's take a closer look at how some of the major players in this immune power drama act out their parts. We've even arranged them in alphabetical order so that you can flip back to them while you're reading the rest of this book.

Antibodies. Antibodies are the weaponry of your body's immune system. Deployed by the B-cells, these Y-shaped protectors patrol your bloodstream, whipping in between cells, searching for any invading bacterium, virus, or microbe that can make you sick. When they find the invader, they grab it with one of the upper branches of the Y. Their microscopic half nelson effectively neutralizes some invaders – bacterial toxins and viruses, for example.

Antibodies need added help to subdue some other invaders. In that case, the lower branch waves in a chemical warfare expert called complement to do the actual killing.

Although each antibody is custom-tailored by your B-cells to grab a specific invader, there are five general kinds of antibodies: immuno-globulin A (IgA), immunoglobulin D (IgD), immunoglobulin E (IgE), immunoglobulin G (IgG), and immunoglobulin M (IgM).

Monoclonal antibodies, however, are antibodies that are artificially created in the lab. They are produced as a result of a coupling between a type of white blood cell and a B-cell cancer cell. The offspring of this unlikely alliance is a *hybridoma,* a hybrid cell that can produce millions of specific antibodies. It is frequently developed to recognize cancer cells so that it can carry drugs to a specific target such as a tumor.

Antigens. Antigens are anything that your body's defense system per-ceives as an invader. They can be viruses, bacteria, or microbes. They can be chemicals, foods, or dust. Generally each antigen has a unique three-dimensional shape that allows a defending antibody to fit into it the way a key fits into a lock.

Autoimmunity. Autoimmunity occurs when your immune system, instead of defending your body, literally attacks it. It's similar to being mugged by your own shadow. Autoimmunity happens when the lethal components of the immune system – macrophages, neutrophils, T-cells, antibodies – can't tell the difference between "self" and "not-self." Instead of destroying only the not-self, these little warriors attack the self, too. The result can be suicidal. There are at least 28 recognized diseases that are caused by such self-inflicted attacks. Some are localized diseases such as myasthenia gravis, a muscle weakness that often develops in the face and can result in drooping eyelids. Some are system-wide diseases such as systemic lupus erythematosus, which can affect the body's collagen. Targets can be the tissue lining of joints, resulting in rheumatoid arthritis, or the myelin sheath around nerve fibers, causing multiple sclerosis. Treating an autoimmune disease is a balancing act, using drugs and radiation to suppress the immune response yet allowing it to continue to function well enough to protect against infection.

B-cells. B-cells are the admirals of your body's defense system. They deploy the antibodies into your bloodstream and other body fluids. They also keep the war records of previous battles so that any invasion by a former foe is immediately countered. In a return engagement, the enemy never even penetrates your defense systems enough to make you sick.

Bone marrow. Bone marrow is the cradle of immunity and the number one immune system organ. It is the source of stem cells, which are the forerunners of a wide variety of immune system cells. Marrow is the place where stem cell genes are rearranged so that they eventually become these immune cells. By adulthood, immunity-producing marrow is found only in the flat bones of the skull, breastbone, ribs, spinal column, collarbone, upper arm, and thigh. When the body needs more white cells to fight an infection, the marrow can immediately speed up the assembly line. Along with the thymus, bone marrow is a primary lymph system organ. But in adults it's also a secondary lymphatic organ because it stores mature T-cells and antibody-producing B-cells.

Central nervous system. The central nervous system contains your brain and spinal cord. Historically, scientists thought that the central nervous system was totally separate from the immune system. Now they're beginning to believe that the two systems communicate through chemical messengers. In fact, some of those messengers – hormones produced by the thymus – are being studied as possible tools to treat and correct a number of brain diseases.

Complement system. Complement is a series of proteins – molecules of carbon, hydrogen, oxygen, and nitrogen – that are called in by an antibody to destroy an enemy. They fall into formation one at a time on the enemy's surface. When the last protein is in place, the complement punctures the enemy's protective coating, allowing its guts to spill out. Then it signals the macrophages and neutrophils to come in and mop up the mess.

Gamma globulin. Gamma globulin is a concentration of antibodies that is separated out from the blood of a donor. It can then be injected into someone who has been exposed to a disease like hepatitis, measles, mumps, whooping cough, smallpox, diphtheria, or chickenpox. The shot provides short-term protection. It's also used to protect children who lack antibodies or complement because of a genetic defect, and it can protect the unborn children of women with Rh-negative blood. Recently gamma globulin has been used to prevent life-threatening infections in children with AIDS (aquired immune deficiency syndrome). In one study, for example, 12 of 14 AIDS-infected infants treated intravenously with gamma globulin survived, while only 14 of 27 who were not treated made it without the serum.

Helper T-cells. *See* T-cells.

Hormones. Hormones are chemical messengers that relay instructions from endocrine glands – the hypothalamus, pituitary, or thymus, for example – to other parts of your body. Some hormones suppress the immune system, others stimulate it. In particular, steroids and corticosteroids from the adrenal glands are known to interfere with the way T-cells do their jobs. Thymosin, a hormone produced by the thymus, is known to help them.

Hybridoma. *See* Antibodies.

Immune complexes. Immune complexes are the debris left floating around after the complement system destroys an invader. They're literally bits and pieces of antibodies, antigens, and complement.

Immunity. Immunity is a condition that occurs when your body's B-cells remember that a particular invader has attacked you before. The B-cells actually generate antibodies to the invader so fast that you never even know it was around. You were immune to its charms.

Immunodeficiency. Immunodeficiency is a loss of some (or all) of the immune system functions. When a body suffers from immunodeficiency, it can't resist infections. AIDS is such a condition. Immunodeficiency is usually congenital but is sometimes acquired, as with AIDS.

Inflammation. Inflammation is the most effective defense mechanism in the animal kingdom. It is a sign that your immune system is at work. Inflammation occurs at the site of an injury, whether deep inside the body – the lungs, for instance – or on and in the skin. Inflammation usually involves heat, redness, swelling, pain, and loss of function in the injured area. The heat and redness are caused by the flow of blood to the injury. The blood is bringing white blood cells, called leukocytes, to fight infection. In your blood vessels, the walls become more permeable, allowing the leukocytes to pass through them. They then enter the extracellular spaces – the spaces between individual cells. Thus set free, the leukocytes maneuver to trap foreign particles by eating them. If an injury is severe enough, pus will form. Pus is made up of leukocytes and the debris of the immune battle.

Inflammation also has a bad side: If severe enough, it can cause permanent damage to surrounding tissues.

Interferon. Interferon got its name because of its ability to interfere with viral infections. It's manufactured in the body by various types of cells that have been infected by viruses. Interferon can't save the infected cell, but it can sound the alarm to alert other cells. When the virus does arrive at the uninfected cells, they're ready for it and produce antiviral weaponry that keeps the virus from reproducing inside the cell. Thus the cell is saved and the progress of the virus is slowed or stopped.

The new science of gene splicing has created bacteria that can produce several different types of interferons in the test tube. As a result, more of this precious protein is available for study and for use in treatment.

Interleukins. Interleukins are hormones that carry messages from one immune system cell to another. They tell the receiving cell to get busy and multiply because antigen invaders are on the attack.

Of at least five different types of interleukins, interleukin-1 (IL-1) and interleukin-2 (IL-2) are the most studied. IL-1 is produced by a macrophage that has devoured an antigen invader. Its most obvious effect is to cause a fever and induce fatigue and sleep. On a microscopic level, IL-1 attracts a T-cell to its "parent" macrophage like a bee to clover. It then stimulates that T-cell to make interferon and IL-2.

In turn, IL-2 causes massive reproduction of helper T-cells to spur the immune response, gets natural killer cells to pursue and destroy the antigens, and stimulates B-cells to produce antibodies.

Interleukins, especially IL-2, are seen as having great potential as medicines, notably in cancer therapy, and are now being genetically engineered in the laboratory.

Killer T-cells. *See* T-cells.

Leukocytes. Leukocytes are white blood cells, the army of the immune system. They have a vast array of duties, and like an army, they are divided into specialized battalions. However, all leukocytes have two main things in common. One, they move to different parts of the body where they mature into various kinds of soldiers. And two, they can move like amoebas through blood vessel walls to reach the site of an injury or invasion. At that site, they either kill the invader or produce antibodies. Then they mop up after the battle.

There are two main groups of leukocytes. The biggest group – phagocytes – makes up about 80 percent of all leukocytes and includes such cells as neutrophils and macrophages. The smaller group (about 20 percent) becomes lymphocytes and then B-cells and T-cells.

Lymphocytes. Lymphocytes are the elite of immune system troops. Even so, the body makes about one billion lymphocytes a day and at any one time has about one *trillion* lymphocytes gadding about looking for germs to annihilate.

There are two basic kinds of lymphocytes. They differ only in their functions, but that difference is profound. As leukocytes, some of the cells migrate to the thymus, where they mature into five different kinds of lymphocyte T-cells. Others remain in the bone marrow to become lymphocyte B-cells.

Lymphokines. Lymphokines are hormones that signal between immune system cells, in effect calling up the troops because the aliens (antigens) have landed. They are produced by lymphocytes and macrophages and include interleukins, interferons, and B-cell growth factor (BCGF).

Lymph system. The lymph system makes up only 2 percent of your total body weight, but it's a couple of pounds you couldn't live without. It produces and deploys the troops that fight off germs, viruses, and allergens. It is divided into primary and secondary sections. The primary section (thymus gland and bone marrow) produces the specialized lymphocytes – T-cells and B-cells – and sends them through the lymph vessels to the secondary organs (lymph nodes, spleen, tonsils, appendix, and a few other organs). These serve as a staging area where the forces of immunity gather in a constant state of readiness to fight the enemy. It is from the lymph nodes that lymphocytes enter the bloodstream. Lymph nodes also have webbed areas that trap antigens and filter them out of the lymph fluid.

Mast cells. Mast cells have been called sentinel cells because they can trigger quick response to an invasion. Although mast cells are related to neutrophils and macrophages, nobody knows exactly what they're for – but they seem to specialize in making people miserable. During an allergic reaction, for example, they release histamine, the substance you take *antihistamines* to control. Mast cells are indirectly responsible for the sneezes, the runny nose, the hives, or whatever little miseries are visited upon you during an allergy attack. One immunologist says mast cells in allergic people are "armed bombs" with the antibody IgE as the firing pin. Contact with an allergen sets the bomb off. On the good side, mast cells may have a role in immunity against parasites.

Mucus. Mucus is, immunologically speaking, your inner skin. This slimy secretion lines lymph system tissues, especially in the "food chute" from mouth to anus, the respiratory tract, and the urogenital tract. All kinds of germs try to enter the body through these orifices, and the mucosal associated lymphoid tissue (MALT) is waiting for them with lympho-cytes and antibodies of all types.

Natural killer cells. Natural killer cells are the Green Berets of immunity. They are another type of lymphocyte closely related to the killer T-cell. But they differ from killer T's in that they're not as picky about what they will or won't kill. They have an innate ability to recognize virally infected cells and some tumor cells and kill them. When they find formerly healthy cells now infected with viruses, bacteria, fungi, or parasites, they produce a chemical that scientists think may poke holes in the cell, thus killing the cell and the antigen.

Neurotransmitters. Neurotransmitters are the chemical messengers of the nervous system. They are secreted from nerve endings to transmit signals from one cell to another. They're also proof positive for scientists that there is a connection between the central nervous system and the immune system. Endorphins, for example, are neurotransmitters that have strong painkilling effects. Called the body's own morphine, they're known for producing the "runner's high."

Researchers have found that white blood cells (in the immune system) have "sockets" that endorphin molecules (from the nervous system) can "plug" right into. Endorphins have an active part in helping white blood cells mature. They've also been found to increase the activity of natural killer cells, a finding that has significance for cancer therapy. And it's been found that lymphocytes themselves can make enkephalin, a relative of endorphins. This fact leads some researchers to think that these chemicals may serve as "intercoms" between lymphocytes, with the central nervous system playing no role. The bottom line is that your nervous system – your emotional state, for example – can have an impact on the state of your immunity.

Other neurotransmitters – acetylcholine, serotonin, and dopamine – have also been shown to affect the immune system in various ways.

Neutrophils. Neutrophils are particularly speedy, hungry, and efficient little scavenger cells whose purpose in life is to swarm all over foreign invaders, swallow them whole (a process called phagocytosis), and kill them with enzymes. A type of white blood cell, neutrophils are also called polymorphonuclear leukocytes. They are produced in the bone marrow faster than Stephen King produces best-sellers – at the rate of 80 million per minute. They live only two or three days. Representing 60 to 70 percent of all leukocytes, they are the first line of defense when an invader breaches the walls of the body – the skin or mucous membranes.

Phagocytes. Phagocytes are any cells that eat and digest foreign particles and invaders, loosely termed antigens. They land like the Marines, arriving in force at the site of an inflammation. They grab the antigens with sticky "hands" that ooze out from the cells' bodies and pull the antigens into their bodies, making a tasty meal of them. The phagocyte family is part of the reticuloendothelial system and includes macrophages, monocytes (precursors of macrophages), and neutrophils. The invaders that they do battle with can be tiny pieces of a wood splinter in your finger, asbestos fibers, bacteria, tumor cells, particles of cigarette smoke or air pollution, pollen, or parasites. Phagocytes also clean up the battlefield after infection skirmishes between immune system troops and aliens. (Phagocytes, however, don't do viruses.) They're so good at what they do that they can even do it on microscope slides and in test tubes as well as in the body.

Phagocytes are found throughout the body, especially in the liver and the lungs. Although phagocytes can usually recognize any foreign particle as an invader, they work best when that particle has been red-flagged by a run-in with an antibody from the complement system. In fact, people whose complement systems are deficient often suffer repeated bacterial infections because their phagocytes aren't readily able to spot invading particles.

One problem with phagocytes is that they sometimes don't seem to know when to stop fighting. As a result, they can do some impressive internal damage. Although they don't actually swallow healthy tissues that border on the battle scene, they continue to produce large amounts of corrosive enzymes, causing diseases like gout, emphysema, asthma, and autoimmune afflictions like rheumatoid arthritis. In fact, phagocytes that have run amok are even implicated in the tissue damage resulting from heart attacks.

Reticuloendothelial system. The reticuloendothelial system is called the RES for short. But it could also be called the phagocyte system or the macrophage system, because it helps manufacture these two immune components. And just because you may never have heard of it doesn't mean it's not important. The RES is found throughout the body. Some RES phagocytes line blood vessels and various organs, becoming mobile only when stimulated by inflammation, while others circulate freely. No alien cell or particle with half a brain wants to get anywhere near an RES cell.

Skin. The skin is more than a big Baggie that keeps your insides from falling on the ground. This largest organ of the body is essential to immunity. It not only keeps the right things inside, it also keeps the wrong things outside. Very few infectious organisms can penetrate healthy, undamaged skin. That's why treatment of cuts, scrapes, and burns is so important. In addition, the skin produces fatty acids that are poisonous to many infectious agents. In fact, some germs' power to cause disease is related to their ability to survive on the surface of the skin.

Spleen. The spleen is a secondary lymph organ best described as a wonderfully discriminating filter of the blood that flows through its meshwork. The spleen helps monocytes mature into those defender warriors called macrophages. It also traps T-cells and B-cells and sorts them into compartments, where they interact with macrophages and antigens for antibody production and other immune functions. People without spleens, or with injured or diseased spleens, get more infections and more serious ones.

Suppressor T-cells. *See* T-cells.

T-cells. T-cells get their name because they are formed in the thymus. The three basic kinds of T-cells are helpers, suppressors, and killers. When put on the alert, a helper T-cell starts dividing into maybe 1,000 identical clones called memory cells. All of these clones remember the antigen that put them on the alert, so anytime that antigen invades the body in the future, it will run into helper T-cells with the memories of elephants.

Helper T-cells also trigger the maturation of B-cells and killer T-cells. Killer T's zero in on cells infected by viruses and on tumor cells. They identify the invading troublemaker, then hunt down any others marauding in the body. They find their victims and bore holes in them with a chemical they secrete. The victim then swells, bursts, and disintegrates. These killer T's continue their search-and-destroy mission until suppressor T-cells call them off.

Thymosin. Thymosin is a hormone secreted by the thymus that helps lymphocytes mature into T-cells.

Thymus. The thymus is one of the two primary lymph organs. It's in the cortex of the thymus that lymphocytes from the bone marrow mature into thymocytes. (Mysteriously, it's also where 99 percent of them die.) Only 1 percent become T-cells and are kept on alert in case of infection. The thymus, located behind the breastbone, reaches its maximum development during puberty but continues to play a major role in immunity for life.

Tumor necrosis factor. The tumor necrosis factor (TNF) is a substance secreted by macrophages, and it is a two-edged sword. TNF is the weapon a macrophage uses to kill tumor cells. Yet it also stimulates the growth of new blood vessels in the tumor, helping the tumor to grow. As the number one secretion of macrophages, TNF is being found to have a major role in inflammation and immune response. And because of its ability to promote the growth of blood vessels, it has a role in wound healing.

Part II
An Immune Power Encyclopedia

3

ADDICTIONS: TOBACCO, ALCOHOL, AND MARIJUANA

Raoul MacGillicuddy has an IQ of 163, but it doesn't seem to help. He likes drinking and smoking so much he named his kids Harvey Wallbanger and Philip Morris. His idea of relaxation is to assume the potato position on the couch with a case of beer on his left and an ashtray on his right. Raoul's relaxation makes him pay the next day with decibel intolerance, pupils that make squeaky-door noises as they constrict, aching hair, and beer-hauling Clydesdales tromping though his head.

Raoul also gets four colds a year, off-and-on bronchitis, and if there's a flu bug flitting around, it will land on Raoul. His cuts don't heal as fast as they should. He misses more Mondays than anyone at work. In addition to all these health troubles, Raoul also had better prepare for what his doctor has warned is probably coming down the pike: liver disease, lung cancer, and an out-of-work immune system.

There's no escaping the facts about alcohol and tobacco. Both can wreak havoc on the immune system. Studies in the test tube, in laboratory animals, and in humans verify the impact these drugs have on the body's ability to fight off invasions. And when they're combined, as they very often are, their ill effects may multiply.

Doctors warn that addictive substances can lead to a variety of health problems.

THE SUBVERSIVE EFFECTS OF SMOKING

Of all the popular drugs, tobacco probably does the most damage to immunity.

Of all the popular drugs Americans take, tobacco probably does the most damage to immunity. About 125,000 Americans die every year of smoking-induced cancer, and another 62,000 succumb to chronic bronchitis and emphysema. You can figure on losing about 5½ minutes of life for every cigarette you smoke. The more and the longer you smoke, the riskier it is. Here are some of the ways your immune system goes up in smoke.

Smoking interferes with the immune system's role in defending the body against tumors caused by viruses.

Smoking hurts your body's ability to fight cancer tumors. The immune system plays a vital part in defending the body against tumors caused by viruses, and smoking interferes with this function. Maybe that's why smokers have higher rates of various cancers, including those of the mouth, lungs, esophagus, pancreas, liver, bladder, ureter, rectum, and cervix. (Some studies have even found nicotine and other tobacco chemicals in cervical mucus!) And while both smokers and nonsmokers can get melanoma – an often fatal form of skin cancer – smokers' melanomas spread throughout the body much more often.

The immune system's cancer-fighting cells aren't as active in heavy smokers as they should be.

If a blood cell can feel any joy in life, one specialized type of white blood cell (the aptly named natural killer cell) finds it by hunting down tumor cells and using a chemical to poke holes in them, which literally makes the tumor cells spill their guts out and die. A University of Kentucky study found these little assassins weren't as active in heavy smokers as they're supposed to be. In fact, their killer cells were only about as active as those in people with lung cancer. The researchers say smoking's effect on killer cells also could be important in the development and spread of tumors.

Smoking upsets the balance of immune power. As in the rest of your body, nature has built a balance into your immune system. Two specialized types of white blood cells – helper T-cells and suppressor T-cells – are supposed to maintain a certain ratio, with helper T-cells switching the immune system on and suppressor T-cells turning it off.

A West German research team says smoking seems to upset the helper/suppressor balance. Among smokers there was a significant *decrease* in the percentage of helpers and an equally significant *increase* in the percentage of suppressors. When all those suppressors work to turn off the immune system, researchers say, a smoker's immunity to tumors can be lowered.

The good, the bad, and the inflamed. Tobacco smoke stuns the small hairs (cilia) in the air passages of the lungs. These cilia act like natural filters, keeping foreign material out of the lungs. In smokers, these hairs become paralyzed, allowing foreign material to enter the lungs – leading to increased infection and inflammation.

White blood cell counts rise whenever and wherever there's an irritation, infection, or tumor. This reaction is called inflammation. Inflammation is a sign the immune system is reacting – and that's good. But excessive inflammation can itself cause damage to cells – and that's bad. Studies show that smokers have white blood cell counts up to 30 percent higher than nonsmokers. Experts say such high counts show that cells have been injured – the kind of injury found in both cancer and heart disease. (In fact, a high white cell count is a strong predictor of heart attack.)

Other studies have found increases of up to 44 percent in a type of white blood cell called neutrophils and fivefold to tenfold hikes in lung

Smoking seems to upset the immune system's regulators, possibly lowering immunity to tumors.

Smokers have white blood cell counts up to 30 percent higher than nonsmokers.

There are also high counts for two immune cells that eat and digest foreign cells.

macrophages. These two immune components are similar in that both eat and digest foreign cells and particles. Such high counts are further evidence of inflammation.

Despite their increased numbers, a smoker's neutrophils don't travel to the battlefield as well as they should, which may explain why smokers get colds and flu more than nonsmokers.

But macrophages in the lungs seem most affected by smoking. This white blood cell's appetite in smokers' lungs seems decreased. That's bad enough, but because they multiply so hugely in smokers, the inflammation they cause is much more likely to damage healthy tissue along with the infected. And such high numbers of macrophages suppress T-cell reproduction in the lungs.

Smoking + macrophages − vitamin E = emphysema. One result of the huge increase in lung macrophages and neutrophils is a glut of waste products produced by these cells. This waste contains oxidants and free radicals, two substances that can cause cell injury, which in turn can lead to disease. But the injury doesn't stop there. Smoking adds an insult – low levels of vitamin E.

Smokers in an Ohio State University study had deficient levels of vitamin E in the fluid that protects their alveoli, the tiny elastic air sacs in the lungs. Vitamin E is an important ingredient of the fluid, as its antioxidant properties disarm the oxidants and free radicals. Without enough vitamin E, the oxidants are allowed free access to the cell membranes, the cells themselves, and the connective tissues. The oxidants cause the cells to become scarred and lose their elasticity, then finally die. The result is an increased risk of emphysema.

Even vitamin E supplements didn't bring levels up to those of nonsmokers. This last point

High counts of immune cells produce a glut of waste products in the lungs that can cause lung cell injury.

Smoking also leads to vitamin E deficiency, resulting in an increased risk of emphysema.

is especially important to Ohio State University researcher Eric Pacht, M.D., who issued this advice: "The worst thing smokers could do would be to take vitamin E and continue smoking. The best thing that could happen is for smokers to stop smoking."

Meanwhile, deep down in the bowels . . . Italian researchers say they've found "clear evidence" that smokers have a higher risk of getting Crohn's disease, a severe, chronic inflammation of the bowels. The inflammation is accompanied by impairment of the immune response, although it's not known which comes first, immune impairment or disease.

Smokers have a higher risk of inflammatory bowel disease.

How not to compromise your infant's immunity. When a pregnant woman smokes, she quadruples her baby's risk of developing allergies. A Swedish study found that the babies of parents *without allergies* were the most susceptible. Smoking hikes the amounts of the antibody immunoglobulin E (IgE) threefold. IgE antibodies sensitize cells in the mucous membranes and skin, causing them to react to allergens by producing rashes, hives, hay fever, asthma, or anaphylactic shock. That IgE increase gives an infant four times as great a chance of developing allergies before 18 months of age as the child of a nonsmoking mother. Another study showed 70 percent of smokers' infants with elevated IgE levels developed allergies before they were 18 months old and 85 percent before they reached 7 years old.

When a pregnant woman smokes, she quadruples her baby's risk of developing allergies.

Can you undo the damage? "Smoking is a two-pronged assault," says Wayne Vial, M.D., a pulmonary specialist in Charleston, South Carolina. "Not only does it increase the likelihood for you to develop malignant cells, it also decreases the likelihood for you to be able to deal with them." Some of the ill effects of smok-

Some of smoking's ill effects can be reversed by quitting.

ing can be reversed by stopping, and quitting certainly keeps things – especially emphysema – from getting worse.

"We hear all the time, 'Doc, I've already done the damage, what difference does it make?'" Dr. Vial says. "But there is no 'point of no return.' There are studies that show that people who have lung disease so severe that they have to be on oxygen therapy all the time still benefit by stopping smoking – even at the end stage of their lung disease."

Don't waste your time looking for a substitute for quitting.

Don't waste your time looking for substitutes for quitting – ways to erase the negative effects of smoking even though you continue the habit. "There's no magic bullet for cigarette smoking," Dr. Vial says.

If Dr. Vial has any self-help advice to offer smokers, it's this: "Quit."

ALCOHOL SUPPRESSES IMMUNITY

Alcohol is a unique and effective immune suppressant.

Alcohol by definition is a toxic drug. It harms the entire body, not just your head and stomach. It adversely affects almost every biological system, including immunity. Alcohol, in fact, is a unique and effective immune suppressant. Pathology professor David Kaplan, M.D., Ph.D., of Case Western Reserve University's Institute of Pathology, says that alcohol's method of suppressing T-cells is so effective that a drug with this ability (but without alcohol's toxic effects) would be a useful tool to combat unwanted immune responses.

Alcohol can be damaging even at low levels.

Most research on alcohol's effect on the human immune system has been conducted with alcoholics. Very little research has been done on the effects of light or even moderate drinking. "But there's so much evidence that alcohol is damaging to the immune system at high levels, there's every reason to think it's damaging even at low levels," says Ronald R. Watson, Ph.D., research professor with the University of Arizona Department of Family and Community Medicine.

Studies of alcoholics show they have higher risk of infection, cancer, and liver disease. Alcoholism has been shown to alter the immune system's response to challenges by preventing a wide variety of white blood cells from working properly. In addition, alcoholics' bone marrow sometimes doesn't produce enough neutrophils. One study also showed that the few neutrophils alcoholics *did* have didn't move as well as they should to the site of infection. Alcoholics with alcoholic liver disease also have T-cells that don't function well. Moreover, their macrophages are on reduced power as they try to clean bacteria from the lungs, liver, and peritoneum (the membrane lining the walls of the abdominal and pelvic cavities). This impaired function helps to explain why alcoholics get pneumonia so easily, according to Rob Roy MacGregor, M.D., of the University of Pennsylvania School of Medicine.

Alcoholics have a higher risk of infection, cancer, and liver disease.

Alcoholics also commonly don't have enough zinc or vitamin B_6 in their bodies. Unfortunately, vitamin B_6 is probably the most important B vitamin for proper immune function, according to Alan Gaby, M.D., author of *The Doctor's Guide to Vitamin B_6*.

But you don't have to be an alcoholic to suffer the adverse effects of alcohol on your immune system. Almost all studies of alcohol and cancer associate a 40 to 60 percent higher risk of breast cancer with even *moderate* drinking, according to the *New England Journal of Medicine*. Women who are obese, have had few children, who were first pregnant after 25, or whose mothers had breast cancer are at especially high risk, the journal says, and should curtail their drinking.

Even moderate drinking may lead to a greatly increased risk of breast cancer.

Moderate drinking can stimulate the immune system.

There is a flip side to moderate drinking. Charles Mendenhall, M.D., Ph.D., professor of medicine at the University of Cincinnati College of Medicine and chief of digestive disorders at the Veterans Administration Medical Center, found that two mixed drinks a day actually *stimulate* the immune system. "It was very surprising to us," he says. "Maybe there's something to the old wives' tale that if you have a cold, take a hot toddy and go to bed and get lots of rest."

But this benefit lasts only a week in animal studies. "If you keep drinking, the immune response appears to go back to normal," Dr. Mendenhall says. "Continued drinking, say for a month, may suppress the immune system."

Binge drinking suppresses the immune system.

Bingeing is out, too. "Immune suppression is almost immediate (within 48 hours) with a large dose of alcohol," Dr. Mendenhall says, "so binge drinkers who go out drinking on a weekend probably put themselves at risk."

The message seems obvious. If you drink, drink lightly, and be sure to eat a varied diet. Don't make things worse by smoking. Don't binge. If you do drink, beta-carotene or vitamin A supplements may boost your probably depleted immunity. Sufficient exercise has also been shown to boost tired immune systems.

MARIJUANA AND IMMUNITY

Studies about marijuana's impact on the immune system are contradictory and controversial.

The debate about marijuana's impact on the human immune system is ongoing. Studies are contradictory and, according to marijuana researcher David Ou, Ph.D., "very controversial." The fear is that the ingredient that gets pot smokers high, tetrahydrocannabinol (THC), may also lower their immunity.

Dr. Ou, clinical assistant professor of pathology at the University of Illinois and chief of immunology at the Veterans Administration West Side Medical Center in Chicago, does his research using pure THC in the test tube and in laboratory animals. Although his results cannot be translated directly to the human body, they're worth looking at.

- Macrophages are supposed to move quickly to gobble up invading microbes. But THC cuts their ability to move to the sites of invasion.
- Once macrophages attach themselves to the invading microbes, they're supposed to start eating the bad guys. But THC substantially decreases their ingestion capability. Dr. Ou is now looking at how well THC-affected macrophages actually kill the microbes they eat.
- High levels of THC suppress the immune response of lymphocytes.
- Under THC's influence, certain body organs, such as the spleen (which is essential for maintaining an effective defense) may shrink in size.

In laboratory animals, THC has a number of effects on immune functioning.

Other researchers have found adverse effects in humans and animals, Dr. Ou notes. They've found that the structures of lung macrophages, neutrophils, and other white blood cell types are altered in chronic hashish users, and that THC and marijuana extracts inhibit the immune response of rodents and interfere with their resistance to herpes simplex virus infections.

But there have been no studies of longtime pot users that link increased disease to decreased immunity. Even with the test tube findings, researchers stress that the effects seem to depend upon the dose and that they are reversible if pot use is stopped. "I don't have hard evidence that THC has the same effects on the body as in the test tube," says Dr. Ou. "But if THC damages

There are no studies linking longtime pot use to decreased immunity.

monocytes in test tube studies, it's probable that marijuana has a bad effect on the immune system."

Dr. Ou says the occasional pot smoker probably wouldn't build up enough of the drug in the body to show the effects he's found in the test tube. It might be different for the heavy pot smoker. And to stop smoking would have a beneficial effect immediately.

THE EVIDENCE IS CLEAR

Addictive behaviors have a definite impact on human immunity.

Perry Mason would have no trouble finding the real killers of a human immune system. As he concisely enumerated the facts and entered them into evidence from exhibit A through Z, Lady Nicotine, John Barleycorn, and Mary Jane would finally stand up in court and cry, "Okay! I confess! I did it! I killed immunity! But I didn't mean to! This wasn't supposed to happen! It wasn't our fault! We were just having a little fun."

So you want to have a "little fun." Putting your immune system on self-destruct may be fun in the short run. But life is risky enough without taking unnecessary chances with the thing that keeps you alive: your immune system. Think about it. The longer you live, the more fun you can have.

4

AGING:
BUILDING IMMUNITY
INTO OLD AGE

Edna Thulin Watts handles Florida real estate worth hundreds of thousands of dollars, sits on the governing body of a 1,100-member church, walks 2 miles a day, and travels to Spain, Hawaii, Alaska, Mexico, or wherever her curiosity takes her. Edna Thulin Watts is 71. And she wears black lace negligees to bed.

Irv Hollingshead is a little younger. Irv, a retired professor of mathematics at Kutztown University of Pennsylvania, is 60. As regional head of a political action group, Irv spends much of his time stopping people on the street to sign petitions, lobbying his congressional representatives in Washington, and demonstrating his personal philosophy by the roadside of the Fortune 500 company that manufactures guidance systems for nuclear warheads. He is a member of the oversight committee of his local Quaker meeting and – unless he's networking in Boston or politicking in Washington – he rarely misses a morning run along the roads near his 18th-century farmhouse.

Statistically these people are old. But are they really? Old is supposed to be rocking chairs, rheumatism, Geritol, catarrh, and constipation. But is it?

Increasingly, it seems, it's not. Increasingly, it's more like Claude Pepper telling off the entire U.S. Senate. It's Katharine Hepburn filming a

Many elderly people manage to remain vibrantly active in their later years.

Statistically these people are old, but their lives tell a different story.

35

New England water scene in 20-degree weather. It's Margaret Thatcher dispatching a fleet of ships to the Falklands. Or Linus Pauling telling a blue-ribbon panel of scientists to go back to their test tubes and try again.

Even the television images of "old" have changed. Twenty years ago the late Walter Brennan played Grandpa McCoy as a gimpy, cantankerous old man whose impaired reasoning required delicate handling. Today, television's old men are chasing crooks, while its old women – armed with a formidable intelligence and a pair of false eyelashes – are catching them.

What's happening to "old?" It's beginning to disappear – or at least to be postponed. And it's not just because of hair dye and wrinkle cream.

THE NEW OLD

The average human life span has expanded greatly since the days of ancient Rome.

Better diets, better public health measures, and better antibiotics and vaccinations to manipulate or help the immune system against a host of diseases have not only pushed back what we traditionally think of as the infirmities of "old age," they also have expanded the average human life span from 22 years in the days of ancient Rome to 76 years in 1980.

An aging immune system is one of the factors that prevents us from reaching our potential life span.

And we still haven't reached our potential. "Most scientists generally believe that the average maximum life span is around 115 years," says Robert W. Gracy, Ph.D., chairman of biochemistry at both North Texas State University and Texas College of Osteopathic Medicine. But we never seem to make it. Our immune system ages right along with the rest of us and leaves us open to the tumors and infections that can result in ill health and death.

By the time we reach our sixth decade, our T-cells' functioning is significantly reduced.

How does our immune system break down? By the time we reach our sixth decade, explains James O'Leary, M.D., Ph.D., an assistant professor at the University of Minnesota Medical School, the function of T-cells in our bodies that are responsible for shooting down cancers, viruses, bacteria, and other foreign invaders is significantly reduced. And the organ responsible for making these cells – the thymus – is a remnant of our youth.

"A weak thymus means your body doesn't make any new T-cells," says Dr. O'Leary. And the ones you've got are wearing out. In fact, their ability to respond to invaders is almost cut in half.

A REASON FOR AGING

"Some scientists think that this functional decline isn't all bad," adds Dr. O'Leary. "The idea is that the system becomes less active for a reason – to avoid self-destruction.

"As cells age, they lose their ability to tell self from nonself," he explains. You from not-you, tumor cells from lung cells, virus-infected brain cells from healthy brain cells. And neutrophils and macrophages, which are responsible for mopping up after an infection, might not be as careful as they once were. They might destroy the good parts of you along with the bad – as in arthritis.

"Since the system becomes more error-prone, you wind up with fewer problems if it's toned down a bit," says Dr. O'Leary. "Maybe it's something that *should* happen."

Maybe. Or maybe we should figure out how to maintain the immune system at a younger – stronger – level. Especially since it seems entirely possible to do so.

BUILD AN IMMUNE LIBRARY

The key, says William H. Adler, M.D., chief of clinical immunology at the National Insitute on Aging, is to build up your immune system the way you would a library. One "book" is proper nutrition – adequate protein, vitamin A, green

Diet manipulation can affect both life span and the immune system.

vegetables, less fat, more fiber. A second "book" might be learning how to control stress. A third is an annual flu shot starting at age 50, and a fourth, some doctors think, is a diet rich in nutrients but low in calories.

"It's quite clear in rodents that you can manipulate the life span – both the average life span and the maximum life span – by fooling around with diets," says Dr. O'Leary. "The major factor is dietary restriction. If you allow rodents to eat what they want, their immune systems decline. If you undernourish the animals (by restricting calories) without them missing any important nutrients, they live longer."

Animals on calorie-restricted diets develop fewer cancers.

They also seem to live better, reports Roy L. Walford, M.D., a professor of pathology at the UCLA School of Medicine. In one study he conducted, for example, 50 percent of fully fed mice developed cancers of one sort or another, but only 13 percent of the mice on restricted diets did. And other studies seem to indicate that animals on restricted diets also have fewer cataracts and less dry skin, kidney disease, and heart disease.

A low-calorie diet may rejuvenate the human immune system.

How does this translate into human terms? Many scientists aren't sure. But Dr. Walford, who has conducted much of the research in this area, is not willing to wait until the scientific verdict is in. He believes that dietary restriction actually rejuvenates the immune system. So, on a gradual basis, he personally began to restrict calories five or six years ago. Today, at age 63, he generally fasts two successive days each week and eats normally, nutritiously, and fully the other five days.

KEEP AN EYE ON YOUR LYMPHOCYTES

One of the most useful "books" you can add to your immune system "library," however, is lymphocyte monitoring, says Dr. Adler. Keeping an eye on lymphocytes, which are converted into T-cells in the thymus, is important.

Why? "In one study we did, we found that the number of lymphocytes declined three years before a patient died," says Dr. Adler. And it didn't matter whether the patient died from heart attack, pneumonia, cancer, or influenza. Three years from that lymphocyte drop they were dead.

Blood tests may reveal a decline in immune system functioning.

"It could be that your immune system knows when something's about to go bad, even if the rest of you doesn't," guesses Dr. Adler. "Even if your annual medical checkup shows nothing."

How do you detect such a drop? "Look at the lab slip next time your doctor orders a blood test," Dr. Adler suggests. "Take the 'percent of lymphocytes' times your 'white count.' That gives you the number of lymphocytes per milliliter of blood." Then keep a record of each test so you can detect any change, or ask your doctor to do it.

Keep a record of the number of lymphocytes per milliliter of blood.

Don't expect a big change, however. The actual number of lymphocytes isn't what's important – it's the drop. "The changes in our studies weren't something that a doctor would raise his eyebrows at," says Dr. Adler. "They were gradual – within normal limits."

But what good does it do to know you're going to die within three years? Rather than using it as a predictor of death, says Dr. Adler, it can be used as an indicator of danger. You can use it as a kind of early warning system and go hunting for the problem. You can ask your doctor to order a computerized axial tomography (CAT) scan or a positron emission tomography (PET) scan and take a closer look. (Be warned, however, that these tests can be expensive.) Maybe he can figure out what's wrong. Maybe together, you and your doctor can fix it.

A drop in the count can be used as a kind of early warning system.

Trygve Tollefsbol, D.O., Ph.D., an assistant research professor of medicine at Duke University, agrees. He also predicts that we'll be able to solve some of these problems – and those of aging – by tinkering with the immune system itself.

New scientific tools may make it possible to manipulate the immune system.

"The tools are just becoming available in recombinant DNA [DNA from more than one species that is broken up and spliced together in a laboratory]," says Dr. Tollefsbol. "They're allowing us to look for the aging gene – or genes – in the immune system. Then maybe we can manipulate it."

What does this mean to us? Within the next 50 years, predicts Dr. Tollefsbol, we may have to decide how long people should live. And when they should die.

5

AIDS: PROTECTING YOURSELF

AIDS reads like the screenplay for a Grade B movie:

Flash to the big city. Scenes of homosexuals wasting away and dying of a mysterious cause. Intense investigation unearths an incurable disease spread by sex and contaminated blood. The disease mushrooms into an epidemic, threatening the general public. Overnight America's love affair with casual sex comes to an end. And the nation turns back toward traditional values. Monogamy is once again enshrined . . .

If you had handed this plot to a movie producer back in 1979, you would have been laughed off the lot.

A decade later, nobody's laughing. Today, we're all living in the midst of this unlikely scenario, trying to come to grips with the reality of a sexually transmitted disease that kills people.

This unlikely plot—a sexually transmitted disease that kills people—is all too real.

AIDS is a scary disease. And in a lot of ways, it's still a mystery. Scientists, working around the clock, are still trying to get a handle on what makes the AIDS virus tick. They can't get rid of it once it gets into the body, and they haven't been able to formulate a vaccine to stop it in its tracks.

But researchers do know a lot about AIDS and the virus that causes it. What they know can prevent you from getting AIDS. There is no vac-

Your behavior and lifestyle can help protect you from the AIDS virus.

cination that offers protection from AIDS, but your behavior and lifestyle can inject a measure of safety.

IMMUNITY UNDER ATTACK

AIDS is a contagious, as yet incurable disease that attacks the immune system.

The acronym AIDS stands for acquired immune deficiency syndrome. It is a contagious, as yet incurable disease that attacks the immune system.

The immune system is your defense against disease. Billions of white blood cells patrol your body on the alert for enemy intruders. Your immune system attacks bacteria and viruses and kills them, usually before they can make you sick. When your immune system finds isolated cancer cells in your body, it seeks to destroy them before they can grow into tumors. Your immune system is very good at what it does, or you would not be alive. In fact, you need it in order to stay alive.

The AIDS virus attacks helper T-cells.

Now picture the virus that causes AIDS, the human immunodeficiency virus (HIV). It is not your typical germ. Instead of trying to slip past the immune system's defenses, it seeks out cells of the immune system. The AIDS virus attacks a category of T-lymphocytes known as helper T-cells. It uses the material inside these cells to reproduce itself and in the process kills the cells.

"In the late stages of AIDS, the helper T-cells are lost. Early on, there are probably other cells of the immune system the virus targets, namely the macrophages. Whether that precedes the infection of the T-lymphocytes or vice versa is still being defined. We do know that the virus ends up in the T-cells," explains John Leonard, M.D., medical staff fellow with the National Institutes of Allergy and Infectious Diseases and author of *Questions and Answers on AIDS*.

The helper T-cell helps the immune system to do its job.

So, what's so important about the helper T-cell? There are, after all, all kinds of cells in the immune system. The helper T-cell does what its name implies; it *helps* the immune system to do its job. The helper T-cell tells the rest of the immune system when to mount a defense and how big a defense is needed. You might say it issues the call to arms.

Dr. Leonard says he has heard the helper T-cell compared to the conductor of an orchestra. Without the helper T-cell conducting the immune system orchestra, the other players don't know what they're supposed to do.

That's why people who have AIDS get sick with things like pneumonia. That's why they succumb to rare forms of cancer. Their immune systems can't fight back because they're already knocked out.

AIDS NUMBERS MOUNTING

AIDS was first recognized as a disease in 1981, the year the Centers for Disease Control (CDC) began monitoring its ghastly progress. At first a small number of homosexual men in the large coastal cities of America were found to have the disease. More than 90 percent of the people who had AIDS in 1981 have since died from the disease. At the time of this writing, more than 70,000 cases of AIDS have been reported to the CDC. More than 50 percent of these people have died.

AIDS has killed thousands of Americans and is spreading fast.

The CDC estimates that between 1 and 1.5 million Americans are already infected with the AIDS virus and that 30 percent of them will have AIDS by 1991. Clearly, the disease is spreading fast.

Will it brush near you and your family?

C. Everett Koop, M.D., former surgeon general of the United States, has assured us that it will: "*We are not able to control AIDS.* I want to make this point with as much emphasis as possible because, unfortunately, there are still people

The surgeon general of the United States has warned that the threat is real.

in this country, including some physicians, who insist that AIDS is a false scare or a problem limited to homosexuals and I.V. drug abusers. That attitude is dangerous."

Dr. Koop wrote this in a special report published in *Modern Medicine,* a professional publication for physicians. In the report he went on to warn that "No matter where you live, whether it be in a high- or low-prevalence area, AIDS is no longer 'possibly' headed in your direction. It has probably arrived already, and you are likely to see more of it than any of us at this time can know."

Dr. Koop is not talking to the general public in this report. He is warning fellow physicians to brace themselves for treating an onslaught of people suffering from AIDS.

Educating yourself about AIDS is a matter of life and death.

What we can gather from Dr. Koop's warning is that no matter where you live, educating yourself about AIDS is a matter of life and death.

BLOCKING THE AIDS VIRUS

The good news concealed at the center of this horror is that the AIDS virus is a wimp.

That might sound like a bald-faced lie, considering how many people it has killed in the past few years. But compare it to the viruses that cause influenza and the common cold. Cold viruses are tough. Cold viruses fly through the air on sneezes, or make the arduous journey from one human body to the next via a handshake or an improperly washed coffee cup.

The AIDS virus can't survive for long outside the body.

Not so with AIDS virus. The AIDS virus can't survive for long outside the body. It doesn't hang out on toilet seats or dirty dishes. You won't get it from a doorknob, a coworker's sneeze, or a crowded subway car. It won't fly in through your window riding on a mosquito.

You can't get AIDS through casual contact.

"Because you can't get AIDS through casual contact, you can touch somebody with AIDS.

You can shake hands. You can give them a hug. You can even give them a dry kiss on the cheek," explains AIDS consultant Anne Jordheim, Ed.D., chairperson of community health at St. Joseph's College in Brooklyn.

"You can live with a person who has AIDS for years – and people have done that – without contracting AIDS. You can't get it through casual contact or through restaurants or through working together or anything like that. Otherwise, we'd all have it by now."

Health authorities say the AIDS virus is transmitted in three basic ways: through sex with an infected person, through needles shared by drug abusers, and when infected women give birth to infants who are infected.

The AIDS virus is transmitted mainly through sex or when drug abusers share needles.

Before 1985, some people, mainly hemophiliacs, got AIDS from transfusions with contaminated blood. The nation's blood supply is much safer now that blood donors are screened and donated blood is tested for the AIDS virus.

It is still remotely possible for some contaminated blood to get through the screening process despite all precautions that are taken. If you are planning to have elective surgery, ask your doctor about the possibility of banking your own blood.

It is, by the way, safe to donate blood. The needles used to take blood are always new.

SAFE, SAFER, SAFEST SEX

The two key ways of protecting yourself from AIDS are:

Don't have sex with a person who is infected with the AIDS virus.

- Don't have sex with a person who is infected with the AIDS virus.
- Don't share needles with a drug abuser.

It's as simple, and as complex, as that.

How do you know whether your sex partner is infected with the AIDS virus? The danger comes from assuming that AIDS is something that happens only to *them*. Although most of the AIDS cases reported in America so far are among homosexual men (there are very few cases among lesbians), AIDS is by no means confined to homosexuals.

AIDS is spreading into the heterosexual community.

"If you ask if AIDS is spreading into the heterosexual community, the answer is yes," warns Dr. Leonard. "Is AIDS *accelerating* its spread into the heterosexual population? The answer to that is, yes, but slowly.

"It's hard to know how to present this information most responsibly, in a social sense. Because if you actually state what the chances of infection are, the numbers are very low in the heterosexual population. If you qualify that still further by looking at the the chances of infection in one encounter, it almost makes it seem like one can forget about risk altogether. But when you take that low risk and apply it to a large population – all the heterosexually active people in the United States – it means that every day people get infected with the virus."

It is possible to get AIDS from *one* unprotected sexual encounter.

Even though the chances of getting AIDS through heterosexual sex are still quite low, the picture is gradually changing. The more sexual encounters, the more sexual partners one has, the greater the chances of coming in contact with the AIDS virus. It is possible to get AIDS from *one* unprotected sexual encounter with an infected person.

You hear a lot about "safe" sex. It is safe to have sex with a person who is not infected with the AIDS virus, but how can you ever be totally sure?

"The trouble with the AIDS virus," says Dr. Jordheim, "is you can't ask somebody, 'What have you been doing in the last 15 years?' It goes back that far. Then comes the drug situation. 'Have you been on drugs? Have you exchanged needles?' Nobody's going to tell a partner unless they know them very well, and even then maybe they won't tell them."

Couples who practice monogamy are not in danger of getting AIDS through sex, provided they have been faithful to each other for the past several years, according to the surgeon general's Report on Acquired Immune Deficiency Syndrome. Both heterosexual and homosexual couples can protect each other from AIDS by remaining faithful to each other.

Monogamous couples are not in danger of getting AIDS through sex.

Some people are riskier sex partners than others, warns Dr. Jordheim. You are at greater risk of coming in contact with the AIDS virus if you have sex with a man who has had sex with another man since 1977, a drug abuser, a person who frequents prostitutes, or anyone who has sex with multiple partners.

Certain sex partners and sexual practices are more dangerous.

Just as some people are riskier sex partners than others, some sexual practices put an individual at greater risk of coming in contact with the AIDS virus. The idea behind safe sex is to avoid contact with fluids from the body of one's sexual partner. The AIDS virus has been found in blood and semen and, in smaller concentrations, in vaginal fluid, tears, and saliva.

Anal intercourse, with or without a condom, is thought to be especially dangerous. But AIDS can also be transmitted through oral sex and vaginal intercourse, Dr. Jordheim warns.

CONDOMS TO THE RESCUE (MAYBE)

The use of condoms as a barrier may offer some protection against the AIDS virus. But, as anyone who has used them as a means of birth control can attest, condoms are not foolproof. They can leak. They sometimes break. They must be used correctly.

Condoms may offer some protection against the AIDS virus.

Although health officials are recommending the use of condoms to help curtail the spread of AIDS, the evidence for complete protection is certainly not conclusive.

The other side of the coin is that a condom might save your life. If you have sex with a person who is infected with the AIDS virus, that thin membrane could be the only thing standing between you and a sexually transmitted disease that kills, says Dr. Jordheim.

Proper use of condoms is important.

If you opt for condoms, choose the kind made of latex. Condoms made of animal skin can let the AIDS virus through. Any lubricant used with the condom must be water-based. Oil-based lubricants, such as petroleum jelly or vegetable shortening, can cause the condom to break. Using a spermicide that contains Nonoxynol-9 apparently offers some additional protection against the AIDS virus.

Other barrier methods of birth control – diaphragms, cervical caps, sponges – do not offer protection.

DANGERS OF DRUG ABUSE

Illegal drug abusers are in danger of contracting AIDS through shared needles.

Abusers of illegal drugs are in especially great danger of contracting AIDS. The street drugs themselves are not transmitting the AIDS virus. The problem lies in shared needles. When a person who has AIDS uses a needle, some contaminated blood remains in the needle. The next person to use the needle injects the deadly AIDS virus directly into the bloodstream. That's why it is dangerous to have sex with a person who uses intravenous drugs.

The best AIDS protection for a drug abuser is to get help to quit drugs as quickly as possible. Not everyone who wants to quit is able to do so, however.

Drug abusers can protect themselves by sterilizing their needles.

Drug abusers need to know that some street dealers are repackaging used, dirty needles and selling them as new. Drug abusers could protect themselves from AIDS by learning how to sterilize their needles in rubbing alcohol, a solution of water and common household bleach, or by boiling them.

AIDS – STILL A MYSTERY

People who have been infected with the AIDS virus do not always know that they have been infected. You can't tell that they are infected with the virus just by looking at them. And they can be perfectly sincere in telling you that they are safe, because they believe it themselves. But a person with no symptoms at all can still spread the virus around.

People infected with AIDS can spread the virus even if they don't have symptoms.

Once a person has been infected, the median time before symptoms develop is just over eight years, according to Dr. Leonard.

Once the AIDS virus is inside a person, it can manifest itself in a number of different ways.

The AIDS virus shows itself in a number of different ways.

The symptoms of AIDS-related complex (ARC) include fatigue, prolonged fever, sore throat, coughing, night sweats, swollen glands, shortness of breath, diarrhea, purplish spots on the skin, easy bruising, and weight loss. The AIDS virus can also attack the central nervous system and brain, leading to lack of concentration, memory loss, partial paralysis, and mental disorder.

Doctors use the term AIDS specifically to refer to patients suffering from opportunistic infections and cancers that they get because their immune systems are not working properly.

Note that all of these symptoms might be present in other kinds of diseases. Only a health professional can diagnose AIDS or ARC.

TESTING FOR AIDS

If you think you may have been exposed to the AIDS virus, ask your doctor about the HIV test. The test is an indirect method of detecting the presence of the virus. It measures antibodies that the immune system produces in response to the virus. (Researchers don't know why the antibodies don't eliminate the virus.)

If you think you may have been exposed to the AIDS virus, ask about the HIV test.

People who should request the test include men who have had sex with another man after

1977, hemophiliacs and others who had numerous blood transfusions before 1985, prostitutes, drug abusers, and people who have had multiple sex partners. Because pregnant women can pass AIDS on to their babies, some health authorities recommend that people should be tested for AIDS before getting a marriage license.

The HIV test is not entirely reliable. It takes up to 18 months following exposure to the virus for the test to come out positive, and there are still many false-positives.

Anyone who tests positive is considered contagious.

Anyone who tests positive is considered to be contagious. They are advised to abstain from sex or, failing that, to let their sex partners know they tested positive and to practice safe sex.

They also need to find a physician familiar with the symptoms and treatment of AIDS.

"It's becoming increasingly clear that probably the majority, if not all, of the people who are infected with the virus will go on to develop either AIDS or some manifestation of HIV-related disease," says Dr. Leonard.

"Why some people may carry the virus for longer than eight years and not develop the disease is not known. Why some people develop the disease in the first six months after exposure is not known. To my knowledge there's been no cofactor that's been definitively shown in any sort of lifelike situation, as opposed to a laboratory situation, to influence the course of the disease. What I'm saying is that once a person is infected, we're not aware of anything that either accelerates or decelerates the progression of that disease."

Until an AIDS vaccine is available, the best preventive is education.

Scientists are working around the clock to find a cure for AIDS. They are racing to come up with a vaccine to prevent AIDS. Until such a vaccine is available, the best prevention for AIDS is education.

6

ALLERGIES: GETTING QUICK RELIEF

Thirty-three thousand feet above the earth, Debbie Birx almost died. The 31-year-old physician and researcher from Walter Reed Army Medical Center in Washington, D.C., was on her way to present a paper at the American Academy of Allergy and Immunology's annual meeting in Anaheim, California. The paper detailed a risky way to halt some of the deadly diseases that attack people infected with AIDS. Her findings would keep people alive.

But Dr. Birx almost didn't have a chance to share her work. Halfway across the country on United Airlines flight 97 from Washington, Debbie Birx had a profound allergic reaction.

There was no warning, Dr. Birx reports. Within minutes of eating a few slices of kiwifruit and a small bunch of grapes from her lunch plate, she began to feel light-headed. Her heartbeat accelerated, nearly doubling its normal rhythm, her blood pressure dropped, and her throat swelled until it almost shut off her air.

Fortunately, the United crew was prepared for just this type of emergency. They administered a shot of epinephrine – a stimulant that increases blood pressure and reduces swelling – and Dr. Birx began to breathe more easily.

But the shot was effective only temporarily. As was the next one. And the next. Six injections later, the DC-10's pilot radioed ahead for an

An allergy researcher almost died of an allergic reaction while on an airplane.

The usual emergency measures failed to help her.

ambulance and prepared to put down at Omaha. Within an hour and a half of her first bite of kiwifruit, says Dr. Birx, she was in an Omaha emergency room, pumped full of steroids and doing fine.

KILLER KIWIFRUIT?

Her immune system reacted to a bit of food as though it were a foreign invader.

How could a few slices of fruit almost cost someone their life? The answer, says Dr. Birx, lies in the way her immune system reacted to the food. When the fruit – the kiwifruit rather than the grapes, she suspects – entered her body, her immune system somehow perceived it as an invader. That error triggered the production of massive quantities of warrior antibodies that were specifically designed to drag the "killer kiwifruit" to the mast cells lining the digestive and respiratory tracts, and also to basophils, cells circulating in the blood. The mast cells and basophils locked onto the immunoglobulin E (IgE) warriors with their attached kiwifruit. They began to emit bursts of chemicals that called in neutrophils and eosinophils to destroy the "invading" food.

Unfortunately, these chemicals – predominantly histamines, prostaglandins, and leukotrienes – caused inflammation, swelling, and constriction of muscles in the air passage as a part of their technique for calling in the troops. And for Dr. Birx, the result was a deadly allergic reaction. The Boston Strangler couldn't have closed her airway more efficiently.

WHY DO WE GET ALLERGIES?

Most of us with allergies experience reactions that are not quite so extreme.

Although the chemical response of an allergic reaction is basically the same in everyone no matter what the allergy, most of us with allergies have a somewhat milder reaction than Dr. Birx. We get a little itching, a stuffy nose, runny eyes, maybe even some sneezing. But not the all-out, life-threatening reaction of an immune system so out of control that it almost destroys the person it's designed to protect. Yet why do we get allergies at all? Why do our immune systems overreact to harmless substances like pollen and kiwifruit?

Scientists don't really know. But they do know that a combination of genetics, timing, and exposure clearly influences the development of an overly sensitive immune system. Ten to 20 percent of us develop allergics, says Max Kjellman, M.D., head of the allergy unit at the University of Linköping Hospital in Sweden. If *both* our parents have allergies, we have a 70 percent chance of following suit. If only one parent has an allergy, somewhere between 30 and 60 percent of us will develop an allergy – probably the same kind as our parent.

Ten to 20 percent of us develop allergies.

But you can't have an allergy without having been exposed to the allergen. And the time immediately after birth and weaning seems to be a time when the human organism is particularly susceptible to that kind of exposure. "Being born or weaned during or immediately prior to the peak season of a pollen increases the risk of sensitization to a particular allergen," says Dr. Kjellman.

You can't have an allergy without having been exposed to the allergen.

"This has been shown for grass, birch, and ragweed allergies," he says. Or if you're exposed to cats or even cow's milk at any time during the first six months of life, you're more likely to be allergic to them than someone who had no exposure in those early months of life.

The studies that demonstrate these ideas are so conclusive, adds Dr. Kjellman, that nurses in Sweden's hospital nurseries are not permitted to give cow's milk to infants without a doctor's prescription.

In addition to exposure, genetics, and timing, there's at least one more factor that influences whether or not you develop an allergy. And that's air pollution.

Air pollution influences whether or not you develop an allergy.

Scientists have been puzzled for years over the apparent increase in allergies throughout the industrialized nations, says Bengt Bjorksten, M.D., professor of pediatrics at the University of Linköping. But they're slowly coming to the conclusion that the increase in allergies is due to the increasing levels of pollution throughout the world.

Air pollution primes your immune system for an allergic reaction.

And, no, it's not that you're allergic to the pollution itself. Instead, air pollution primes your immune system for an allergic reaction, explains Dr. Bjorksten. The pollutants – primarily tobacco smoke, nitrogen dioxide, ozone, and sulfur dioxide – rev up your body's IgE levels so that when an allergen hits your airway or your digestive tract, your immune system is so sensitive that it explodes into an allergic reaction.

Interestingly, however, if you don't have a family history of allergy, the pollutants don't seem to have an allergic effect, says Dr. Bjorksten. That difference in family history may explain why some people are apparently sensitive to various pollutants and others aren't.

"We did a survey of 5,100 children in a couple of communities and, just measuring birch pollen, we found that if you are living with parents who smoke and you've got a family history of allergy, you're in trouble for birch pollen allergy," says Dr. Bjorksten. But if you don't have a family history of allergy, then the smoke – even if it's concentrated in your home by 20th-century building practices – won't trigger an allergic effect.

If your mother smoked while she was pregnant, you have an increased chance of developing an allergy.

The one exception to these "rules" of allergy development is if your mother smoked while she was pregnant. In that case, scientists report, you have four times the risk of anyone else for developing an allergy – whether or not you also have a family history of allergy.

POTENTIAL ALLERGENS – INCLUDING EXERCISE!

What kind of allergies are most common? If you have a family history of allergy, apparently you can become allergic to anything at any time.

You can even become allergic to exercise, reports John Wade, M.D., a former researcher at Harvard Medical School. He's not talking about couch potatoes who don't like to sweat. He's talking about serious collapse. A study he conducted of 199 people who became anaphylactic (the type of reaction Dr. Birx had) as they exercised reveals that 92 percent first experienced itching all over their bodies, 83 percent had hives, 79 percent had swelling, 59 percent had difficulty breathing, and 32 percent experienced cardiovascular collapse.

The study found that although more than half of these people were allergic to other things, they had not come in contact with them prior to the workout that triggered their reactions. People who experienced exercise-induced asthma were eliminated from the study.

So what caused the allergy? "Exercise itself," says Dr. Wade succinctly. Seventy-one percent of the study participants were jogging at the time their IgE levels went nuts and triggered the reaction, 38 percent were doing aerobics, 26 percent were dancing, and 17 percent were swimming, although intensity and duration were more important than type of exercise.

If you're prone to other allergies, says Dr. Wade, avoid aspirin and food 4 hours before you exercise. Or if you've ever had any respiratory symptoms while exercising – swelling, difficulty breathing – always exercise with a friend. If you develop itching and flushing all over your body at any time during your workout, stop what you're doing immediately.

It is even possible to become allergic to exercise.

If you're prone to allergies, it is important to take precautions while exercising.

Allergens can provoke every-thing from hives to life-threatening anaphylaxis.

Other allergens are a little more what you'd expect. In fact, pollens from trees, weeds, and grasses are the most common causes of runny noses and itchy eyes, while animals, stinging insects, house dust, molds, and foods aren't far behind in provoking everything from hives to anaphylaxis.

Food allergies, for example, can cause itching and swelling of the lips, mouth, and throat as the offending food is eaten; nausea, vomiting, cramps, gas, and diarrhea as it pummels the intestines; migraines as it hits your brain; a runny nose, stuffy ears, or bed-wetting as it reaches your nose, ears, or bladder; swelling and hives as its proteins are distributed to your skin; or even – as with Dr. Birx – a constricted airway as it clutches your throat.

A food allergy is more likely to trigger a life-threatening reaction than any other allergy.

Unfortunately, a food allergy is apparently more likely to trigger a life-threatening reaction than any other allergy. A study of 89 people who experienced this kind of worst-case allergic reaction revealed that 64 percent of these reactions were triggered by allergies to foods or food additives.

The foods to which people are most likely to be allergic are eggs, milk, tree nuts, peanuts, whitefish, and shellfish. Peanuts, eggs, and milk are the allergens most often implicated in hives. Peanuts, soy, and beef have been implicated in migraine headaches that begin 4 to 6 hours after eating. And shellfish and peanuts are the most likely allergens to provoke an anaphylactic reaction. Shellfish and peanuts can be so toxic, in fact, that even inhaling the steam from boiling or frying fish has been known to leave someone who has a fish allergy literally gasping for breath.

Doctors recommend that sulfite-sensitive people carry an EpiPen at all times.

Sulfites – preservatives that are frequently sprayed on fresh fruit, shrimp, and vegetables or sprinkled in wine, beer, and Mexican food – have also been implicated in anaphylaxis. They can be so deadly and are so frequently hidden in foods that doctors recommend that sensitive people carry an EpiPen – a spring-loaded syringe containing the medication epinephrine – at all times. You may feel like an overgrown Boy Scout, but the EpiPen can save your life.

Fortunately, people frequently outgrow food allergies. In a study at Johns Hopkins University, for example, 25 percent of the study's participants who were allergic to eggs, milk, soy, wheat, and peanuts lost their allergies one year after the allergen was totally eliminated from their diets. Seventy percent of the study participants who were allergic to a mixed bag of other foods also lost their allergies within a year.

People frequently outgrow food allergies.

An allergy to peanuts, however, can be tricky. Other studies indicate that a peanut allergy is *not* outgrown, even over a long period of time. What's worse, figuring out just what is and what is not a peanut is getting pretty complicated.

Ingredients that you are allergic to can sometimes be difficult to spot.

DISGUISED PEANUTS

There's a new type of nut on the market that can look and taste like either a pecan or an almond. But it's not. It's really a peanut. Or, explains John Yunginger, M.D., a consultant in pediatrics and internal medicine at the Mayo Clinic in Rochester, Minnesota, a "reflavored" peanut. The Food and Drug Administration requires that the nut clearly be identified on any food labels as an imitation nut, says Dr. Yunginger, so you should be safe in stores. But how many times do you see labels when you're eating out? When you visit a friend for dinner, would you even think to worry about the "almonds" sprinkled on your string beans?

Probably not. For that reason, the American Academy of Allergy and Immunology recommends that you tell anyone who prepares food for you – a friend, a waiter, a cafeteria worker, anyone – that you're allergic to a particular food. You should also learn which foods are related to the ones that bother you. If you're allergic to shrimp, for example, you may well be allergic to lobster or even freshwater fish.

Naturally, you should also check the ingredients of any food you buy in stores, says Dr. Yunginger. And learn to be pushy in restaurants. Ask the waiter who swears there aren't any allergens in his chef's secret sauce if he'll still swear to it on your grave.

You need to take your allergy just as seriously. "People have a few minor reactions to something they're allergic to and they get cavalier about carrying medication," says Dr. Yunginger. In one study of 89 people who had had allergic reactions that almost killed them, for example, 50 percent of the people who had been warned to carry an emergency kit failed to do so.

Be aggressive about protecting yourself.

That's suicide, says Dr. Yunginger. It's crazy. So is popping an antihistamine or steroid drug so you can go out and eat whatever you want. Or getting a minor reaction and denying that it could be serious. The phrase, "I'll just wait another 10 minutes and see if it subsides" can be the last one you'll utter.

The only way to deal with a food allergy is to avoid that food.

The only way to deal with a food allergy, says Dr. Yunginger, is to avoid the food that kicks your immune system into hyperdrive. Eating a little bit here or a little bit there will only keep you sensitive, and immunotherapy – injecting small amounts of an allergen to try and desensitize your immune system – doesn't work with food. It causes just as much of a reaction as eating the food itself.

DO-IT-YOURSELF DIAGNOSIS

But don't drive yourself nuts trying to figure out your allergies on your own, adds Dan Atkins, M.D., a researcher at the National Jewish Center for Immunology and Respiratory Medicine in Denver. In a study he conducted, for example, 16 out of 44 people who thought they were allergic to a particular food were not. They wasted a lot of time and effort trying to avoid foods without relieving any of their allergy symptoms, he points out, while the real cause of their problem remained undiagnosed.

What you should do if you suspect you have a food allergy, says Dr. Atkins, is ask your doctor to perform a double-blind food challenge. It's a test where you ingest food capsules, but neither you nor your doctor know their contents.

Let your doctor diagnose food allergies with the proper tests.

You then keep a log of symptoms, so you can determine whether or not a particular capsule seems to trigger them. When the nurse checks her log to see which capsules had the suspected allergen and you check your log to see which capsules provoked symptoms, it should be fairly obvious whether or not you're allergic to a particular substance.

A less expensive way to accomplish the same thing, some doctors suggest, is to have a skin prick test done to see whether or not a minute bit of the food provokes a reaction. You then eliminate any suspect food from your diet and see how you do.

Do *not*, however, challenge yourself at home with a food to which you may be allergic. Most reactions to food challenges will occur within 30 minutes to 2 hours, say doctors at the Cleveland Clinic, and you should be under direct medical supervision during that time in case there's an anaphylactic reaction. You should be particularly careful if you've previously experienced anaphylactic reactions. Sixty-two percent of those who've had one episode, studies indicate, may have another.

It is dangerous to attempt food allergy tests at home.

THE WEED THAT SEEDS

But what about the allergens you inhale? Unlike food allergies, which you can usually *decide* to avoid, you really don't have much choice about what you breathe.

The most common pollen allergy is to ragweed.

The most common pollen allergy – affecting somewhere around 5 percent of the population – is to ragweed, says Philip Norman, M.D., a professor of medicine at Johns Hopkins University School of Medicine. Ragweed is the cute little pollen that travels the airways between mid-August and October and covers the hood of your car when it's parked outside. And the only way to get away from it is to vacation in the western mountains, the southern end of Florida, or the northern tip of Maine.

Ragweed can even trigger asthma.

"For some people, it's like a prolonged cold," says Dr. Norman. "For others, it's worse. They get an itchiness in their nose and eyes, maybe their throat, or a runny and stuffy nose both at once. Some people even get asthmatic. If your sensitivity to ragweed is great enough and you have a tendency toward asthma, it can trigger the disease."

There's a lot you can do to turn off the symptoms of almost any inhalant allergy.

Fortunately, there's a lot you can do to turn off the symptoms of almost any inhalant allergy, says Dr. Norman. You can, for example, spray, inject, or swallow steroid drugs that interfere with the way your body releases the chemicals – like histamines or leukotrienes – that cause the swelling and leaking of eyes, nose, and throat. And a nasal spray – with lunisolide or beclomethasone, in particular – will relieve your symptoms without the worrisome side effects that are often associated with systemic steroids.

You can also use decongestants combined with antihistamines or a drug called cromolyn – either sprayed in your nose or dropped in your eye – that coats your mast cells so they won't release the symptom-provoking histamine quite so easily.

But if you get tired of squeezing, popping, dropping, and squirting during your allergy season – or year-round if you're allergic to something like dust – then maybe you should try immunotherapy.

TURNING YOUR IMMUNE SYSTEM OFF

Immunotherapy – a series of injections of whatever it is you're allergic to – is between 60 and 80 percent effective in turning off your allergy symptoms, says Peter S. Creticos, M.D., associate director of the Johns Hopkins Center for Asthma and Allergic Diseases. It appears to work particularly well when you're allergic to cats; dogs; dust mites; tree, grass, or weed pollens; or certain mold spores.

Immunotherapy is 60 to 80 percent effective against allergy symptoms.

It hasn't always been so effective, however. Years ago the dosages were far too low to be effective, and the extracts – a form of concentrated allergen – were not standardized, says Dr. Norman.

The extracts, in fact, were crude. Drug companies used to buy bags of vacuum cleaner dust from housewives to manufacture house dust extracts for immunotherapy, says Thomas Platts-Mills, M.D., Ph.D., head of the University of Virginia's Division of Allergy and Immunology. So if your doctor gave you "allergy shots" for dust years ago, he could have been injecting anything that was in Mrs. Brown's Thursday morning dust: a little mold, a hair of cat, a smidgen of dog, some crunched-up cockroach, perhaps Mr. Brown's psoriasis flakes. How this extract was supposed to prevent an allergic response to the dust in *your* house – which may or may not have included any of the above substances – is anybody's guess.

Today, extracts used to prepare allergy shots have been, to a large extent, standardized. The same element is going to be in the extract every time, and the concentration of the substance will be the same.

This therapy is much more effective today than it was in years past.

"If you tried immunotherapy years ago and it didn't work, try it again," urges Dr. Norman. "Now it should provide some relief."

DISCONTINUING IMMUNOTHERAPY

You need to try the shots for at least two seasons to determine whether they work.

How long should you try the shots? Give them a whirl for at least two seasons before judging their effectiveness, suggests Dr. Creticos. If they seem to work, your doctor will probably suggest continuing the therapy for three to eight years. Consider stopping if your symptoms improve, but be aware that they may return – requiring you to begin the injections again.

Giving immunotherapy enough time to take effect, however, may be well worth the trouble. Studies with sting allergies, for example, indicate that after five years on immunotherapy, 50 to 90 percent of the people who were allergic to an insect sting had lost their allergies.

Your doctor must do tests to find out when your body can safely discontinue immunotherapy.

To find out when discontinuing immunotherapy is safe for *your* body, says David Golden, M.D., an assistant professor of medicine at Johns Hopkins University, ask your doctor to do a skin test and measure the IgE levels in your blood. When your skin test is negative – and nearly half of all skin tests are after eight years of immunotherapy – and your IgE levels drop to normal levels, you can think about discontinuing therapy. If the IgE levels remain high, adds Dr. Golden, think twice about stopping the shots.

Immunotherapy itself does not usually provoke an allergic reaction.

Fortunately, immunotherapy itself will not usually provoke an allergic reaction. In a study at Fitzsimmons Army Medical Center in Colorado, for example, only 2 percent of 100,000 study participants had any kind of reaction. The reactions included swelling at the injection site, nasal congestion, sneezing, itching, hives, and one fatality, according to the study's director, Richard W. Weber, M.D., chief of allergy and immunology at Fitzsimmons. That one fatality, he adds, taught scientists the one kind of person who should *not* receive immunotherapy: someone whose heart and lungs are functioning so poorly that they can't withstand the trauma of anaphylaxis, should it occur.

Unfortunately, sometimes people don't realize they've got pulmonary problems until they land in the hospital. So just in case there's a serious reaction to the shots, anyone receiving immunotherapy in the United Kingdom is required to wait in their doctor's office for 2 hours after an injection. In Sweden, reports Dr. Weber, people are required to wait for 30 minutes after a shot and to have a pulmonary function test both before and after the injection. If there's a decline in lung function of 20 percent or more after the injection, he adds, the recipient is hospitalized.

Because there are no laws governing this issue in the United States, says Sheldon Spector, M.D., an allergist and asthma specialist at UCLA, you'll have to protect yourself. Even though some doctors allow patients to give themselves their own immunotherapy, don't take the allergy extract and syringe home. If you are on a high-dose regimen, you may be in jeopardy, says Dr. Spector. On the other hand, if the doctor is giving you low-dose diluted extracts in order to avoid any possibility of a bad reaction, you're being ripped off.

Protect yourself by not taking the allergy extract at home.

BEATING YOUR BODY TO THE ALLERGIC PUNCH

Because it may take some time for your immunotherapy to take effect, you'll need some help in the meantime. The way immunotherapy works, explains Dr. Norman, is to *de*crease your body's IgE response to an allergen by forcing your body to produce lots of IgG, an antibody that will block the IgE from releasing its trouble-causing chemicals. Apparently simply introducing the allergen by injection is what provokes the IgG to jump into action. Since it may take several months before your body's IgG antibodies are fast enough to beat IgE to the allergic punch, here are a few tips to keep your allergies in line until immunotherapy does its job.

Keep your allergies in line until immunotherapy does its job.

If you have a dust allergy, take steps to control household dust.

- If you have a dust allergy, advises Dr. Platts-Mills, get rid of as many carpets as you can bear, but especially the one in your bedroom. Cover your mattresses and pillows with a plastic-backed dust cover. Regularly wash your bedding in hot water (130° F). Vacuum your house only once a week. Keep the humidity as low as possible. And although air-cleaning devices with high-efficiency particulate air (HEPA) filters do remove a substantial number of particulates from the air, they don't help people with a dust allergy. The reason is that many people with a dust allergy are actually allergic to the dust mite and its feces, explains Dr. Platts-Mills. The mite never gets pulled into the air cleaner. The sticky pads on its feet allow it to stay hooked in your rugs no matter what, and the fecal pellets don't really stay up in the air long enough for an air cleaner to suck them down.

Find ways to avoid allergens from animals, molds, grasses, and so forth.

- If you have an allergy to animals, a HEPA filter can reduce the amount of allergen in your air by up to 70 percent.
- If you have an allergy to specific grasses or trees, avoid hikes, picnics, and other outdoor activities at the times your doctor indicates the pollen count is highest. Indoors, an electrostatic air cleaner may also be helpful, especially if it's hooked up to your central heating and cooling system.
- If you're allergic to stinging insects, avoid wearing brightly colored or black clothing and don't use hair sprays, perfumes, and lotions. Always wear shoes outside to protect yourself from insects nesting in grass.
- If you're allergic to molds, stay out of the basement and the garage as much as

possible or install a dehumidifier in each area to get rid of the moisture. And don't forget to clean it – some experts say at least once a day. Get rid of your houseplants, think twice about raking and burning leaves, and keep the bathroom clean and well ventilated.

- No matter what you're allergic to, consider eating lots of onions. Walter Dorsch, a researcher at the University of Munich, has discovered a compound that's released when onions are squished – either by a food press or your teeth – that actually reduces the amount of histamine produced by your mast cells.

Consider eating lots of onions.

ON THE FRONTIER

And of course, the best tip of all is to take heart, because one of these days you won't have to worry about any of this at all. Not only is immunotherapy finally beginning to fulfill its potential, but according to Michael Kaliner, M.D., head of the Allergic Diseases Section at the National Institute of Allergy and Infectious Diseases, researchers around the country are working on ways to control mast cell production, shut down your body's production of IgE, and locate a switch that can throw your body out of its natural allergic mode and into a less harmful one.

Hang in there; immunotherapy is finally beginning to fulfill its potential.

Think that's farfetched? In one year alone they've already learned that some allergic reactions can be blocked by a derivative of the ginkgo tree or a common substance in fish oil and that interleukin-3, a messenger from one part of your immune system to another, apparently has something to say about the number of basophils and mast cells your body produces and how much – or how little – histamine is released.

Pieces of a puzzle? You bet. But one with solutions just around the corner.

7

ALZHEIMER'S DISEASE: FINDING NEW HOPE

A 69-year-old man forgot which kind of car he drives.

Sam Alexander stopped in front of the shopping center's restaurant and raised a hand to his forehead. Now where was the car? He shaded his eyes from the sun and scanned the parking lot. At age 69 his eyes weren't as good as they had been. And those white balls of Florida sun bouncing off the chrome-edged bumpers and windshields of a hundred late-model cars weren't helping.

He held up his newspaper to blot out the glare. Now where had he parked his car? Where was the light green T-bird with the dark green roof? Or – wait a minute – wasn't he looking for a Buick? Hadn't he traded the T-bird in for a dark blue Buick with white sidewalls? Or was it a white Cadillac? No, he shook his head, no, he'd bought the blue Buick in South Carolina two years ago and his wife had given him the Cadillac for his birthday last month. But had he sold the Buick? Or was he driving it? Which car was supposed to be in the lot?

How would he get home if he couldn't remember?

A NEUROLOGIC RAPE

Such forgetfulness is *not* normal.

Our culture views forgetfulness as a normal part of aging. But, other than the where-did-I-put-my-glasses kind of forgetfulness that affects

66

us all no matter what our age, forgetfulness is *not* normal. It's one of the earliest symptoms of Alzheimer's disease (AD), a neurologic syndrome that rapes the intellect, strips the mind of the words necessary to define AD's existence or tell about the crime, and buries the intellect's corpse where it can't be found – in tangled masses of nerve cells and lumps of protein deep within the brain.

Having this disease means that someone like Sam Alexander not only forgot what kind of car he owns but has also forgotten how to find out. It will not occur to him to look in his wallet for a car registration card, check his keys for an automotive logo, or even check the parking lot for both the Buick and the Cadillac.

He was suffering from Alzheimer's disease.

It also means that when he seeks help from a nearby barber he knows, he won't be able to explain the problem. He'll gesture to the parking lot and tell the barber he "can't find the thing that goes – you know, the thing that I go home in."

Alzheimer's disease is what folks used to call senility.

TANGLES AND LUMPS

What causes Alzheimer's disease? Nobody knows for sure. One theory is that the tangled nerve cells and lumps of protein characteristic of the disease are caused by an old virus that suddenly becomes active. Another is that it's your brain's response to something toxic in the environment, like aluminum. A third is that it's a natural consequence of an aging immune system. A fourth is that it's too little zinc and too much copper in your diet, or maybe too much coconut oil and too little fish oil. And a fifth is that it's somehow genetic.

Nobody knows what causes this disease, but the immune system plays a role.

"The emerging concept of Alzheimer's disease is that this is more of a *syndrome* than a single disease," says Vijendra K. Singh, Ph.D., a research neuroimmunologist at the Medical University of South Carolina. And of the several possible things that can trigger it, the immune system clearly plays a role.

Clayton Wiley, M.D., Ph.D., a pathologist at the University of California, San Diego, agrees. "Most likely, Alzheimer's is caused by some kind of immunosuppression," he says. "One theory, for example, is that a retrovirus is involved. Retros can get themselves encoded into genetic material and be passed to offspring," he adds. And if that happens, your body's immune system won't be able to tell the difference between the virus and any other cell in your body. It will flourish – tucked away in a cell – effectively hidden from any weaponry deployed by your immune system. It's almost as though your immune system has been programmed to ignore it.

Immunologic factors influence the course of this disease.

That might explain some of the findings uncovered by Dr. Singh and his team of researchers in South Carolina. Of all the various factors that might influence the course of this disease, says Dr. Singh, two are clearly immunologic. And one is an apparent malfunction of the T-cells – those generals that essentially orchestrate every attack made by your immune system. They just don't seem to do their job.

Certain agents that stimulate immune function affect Alzheimer's.

"This told us that there is a possibility of using agents which can stimulate the immune function to affect Alzheimer's," says Dr. Singh. And in fact, that is exactly what he's done. Using various forms of pyrrolidine, a chemical that can stimulate the immune system, Dr. Singh and his colleagues demonstrated both in the lab and in human studies that pyrrolidine could activate the apparently suppressed T-cell function in people affected with Alzheimer's disease.

Moreover, he also found that another compound, dialyzable leucocyte extract (DLE), which is made from donor blood cells, has a similar effect on the other major immunologic component of Alzheimer's: the presence of auto-antibodies circulating in the brain.

ANTIBODIES UNEXPLAINED

Now what causes the immune system to produce antibodies to its own brain cells, nobody has quite figured out. Some scientists think it's a natural consequence of aging. Others – like Dr. Singh – think it's one of the causes of Alzheimer's. What can't be disputed, however, is that DLE seems to have as positive an effect on people with Alzheimer's who have auto-antibodies as pyrrolidine does on people with Alzheimer's who have messed up T-cells.

But "positive" doesn't mean some pie-in-the-sky cure, cautions Dr. Singh. "The improvement that we see is something like a patient's ability to identify a spouse – where before therapy the patient couldn't do it. Or, for that matter, identify an object.

"I remember one case, for example, where I had given a keychain to a patient who could not identify what it was. After our treatment process the patient was able to say, 'Isn't that something you open a lock with or a door with?' "

Clearly, these drugs don't provide a cure. They just pull the patient back to an earlier stage of the disease. But the fact that there's improvement – the fact that there can be a reversal – shows us we're on the right track, says Dr. Singh.

"Most scientists have believed thus far that the cells [affected by Alzheimer's] are dead and that's why there's no memory. Now we are changing that thinking. We believe that, instead of dying, the brain cells of people with Alzheimer's

Treatment shows definite promise.

The brain cells of people with Alzheimer's are possibly suppressed.

are merely suppressed," says Dr. Singh. And what has been suppressed, he adds, can probably be reactivated.

IMMUNOLOGY FROM THE SEA

But not all immunologic agents are found in the lab. In fact, some may be found in your kitchen.

Researchers are trying to figure out the effects of diet on Alzheimer's.

How do we know? Well, Edgar S. Cathcart, M.D., D.Sc., chief of staff at the Bedford Veterans Administration Center in Massachusetts, tells us so. He headed a research team trying to figure out the effects of diet on those lumps of protein – called amyloids – that are characteristically found screwing up the circuits in the brains of those with Alzheimer's.

Fish oils reduce the severity of amyloid deposits in the brains of lab animals.

Using mice, he and his colleagues have discovered that fish oils containing omega-3 fatty acids actually reduce the severity of these amyloid deposits in the brain.

Does this mean that a diet rich in omega-3's can help someone with Alzheimer's? "We need to investigate more," says Dr. Cathcart. But, "If fish oil retards amyloids of one type [mice], it may indeed retard the amyloids of another."

And so there's hope for Sam Alexander and others burdened with this strange syndrome that steals what we value most. With a chemical to stimulate the sluggish immune system, another agent to help counter antibodies that have gone wrong, and a dietary factor that holds the promise of reducing amyloid deposits in the brain, the future for those with AD seems brighter.

8

ANTIBIOTICS: NATURE'S SECRET WEAPONS

Bread mold, frog skin, catfish slime, and water taken from a puddle in the Pine Barrens of New Jersey – these sound like the ingredients for a witch's brew. While this recipe may never bubble in a single cauldron, taken separately the potions work some pretty potent medical magic.

Antibiotics are often made from exotic ingredients.

Each of these unsavory substances is a source of antibiotics, the so-called wonder drugs. You pop a pill and debilitating symptoms disappear overnight. Skin infections clear up. Fever cools off. Antibiotics can certainly *seem* miraculous enough.

Perhaps because antibiotics were so effective against a whole host of bacterial infections, the temptation was there to overuse them. And it is because they *were* overused and misused around the world that we are all paying a heavy price, says Stuart Levy, M.D., president of the Alliance for the Prudent Use of Antibiotics.

FIGHTING BACK BACTERIA

Meet Supergerm. Bacteria used to wither and die at the merest hint of penicillin. Now, if bacteria could laugh, you might hear a collective chuckle next time you try taking the stuff. Oh, penicillin still works. Sometimes. It's just that all of us are increasingly likely to run into what are known as resistant strains of bacteria,

Strains of bacteria capable of resisting antibiotics are rapidly spreading.

strains that have developed in only the last few decades. And just what are these microbes resisting? Antibiotics, that's what. That means trouble.

"It turns out that most of the common, inexpensive, relatively nontoxic antibiotics are ineffective against the majority of common bacterial problems – such as pneumococcal pneumonia, ear infections in kids, venereal diseases, hospital-acquired infections, you name it," says Dr. Levy. "The problem is not only their resistance to the single drug, but we now see a phenomenon of multidrug resistance, where a single bacterium is able to live in the presence of three, four, five, even seven or eight different antibiotics."

Overuse of antibiotics contributes to the problem.

Overuse of antibiotics – using them in an ill-advised attempt to treat viral infections, for example – contributes to the problem. Antibiotics wipe out all of the bacteria in a person's body, the helpful ones as well as the bad ones. The only bacteria that survive are the few that are resistant to the antibiotics. They live to pass on their resistant genes, explains Dr. Levy.

Using antibiotics in animals raised for food also adds to the problem.

Contributing to the problem, he believes, is the widespread use of antibiotics in animals being raised for food. Although the animals' bacteria may not pose a direct threat to man, bacteria do swap genetic information. According to Dr. Levy, there is nothing to prevent resistant strains of bacteria that come from animals from transferring their resistance to the kinds of bacteria that cause *human* sickness.

SEARCHING FOR NEW MIRACLES

Resistant germs are certainly not news to large pharmaceutical companies. Tougher germs call for tougher germ-fighting weapons, and companies that make drugs are literally leaving no stone unturned in the search for new sources of antibiotics.

Squibb Corporation recently announced the development of Azactam, the first truly new antibiotic in years. After searching for ten years in more than 200,000 soil and water samples taken from around the world, they found what they were looking for in a water sample from the Pine Barrens of New Jersey. The water yielded bacteria that produced a substance that became the basis for this new antibiotic. Right there in the scrub pine forests of southern New Jersey.

"We like to say the microbes out in nature are smarter than the chemists," says Scott Wells, Ph.D., a Squibb microbiologist.

Because of microbes' antibiotic-making talents, employees of some drug companies take sterile plastic Baggies on their vacations so they can scoop up soil samples for analysis. They never know just where the next antibiotic will be found. Meanwhile, other researchers are out at sea, expanding the search even farther.

"If you look at the classical drug discoveries, they've all been made on land. The ocean hasn't been done before. It's wide open," says Ross Longley, Ph.D., immunologist with Harbor Branch Oceanographic Institute in Fort Pierce, Florida.

The institute's ships ply the seas collecting samples of sponges, corals, and other sea creatures. The organisms are then examined for new sources of antibiotics and other pharmaceuticals that might enhance or suppress the immune system. Their search has been rewarded with several new antibiotics that are now in the testing stages.

New antibiotics are good news for people who are allergic to existing antibiotics such as penicillin. A person who is allergic to one type of antibiotic might be able to tolerate another kind.

Antibiotic actually means "against life," says Dr. Longley. Antibiotics are toxic substances that microbes use against other microbes. Bacteria

Drug companies leave no stone unturned in the search for new sources of antibiotics.

The search is carried out on land and at sea.

Antibiotics are toxic substances that microbes use against other microbes.

competing for territory may secrete a substance that will kill off all the other bacteria in the area – that would be an antibiotic. When we use antibiotics, we are borrowing the bacteria's weapons to bolster the fighting power of our own immune systems.

USING ANTIBIOTICS WISELY

Brand-new antibiotics are all well and good, but in the meantime, what about the old standbys? Is there anything we can do to use antibiotics more wisely? What can we as individuals do to protect ourselves from resistant bacteria?

The Alliance for the Prudent Use of Antibiotics exists to deal with just those issues, and Dr. Levy was more than happy to provide detailed information.

Out with the old. First, check your medicine cabinet. You remember that bottle of antibiotics left over from your spouse's dental surgery last year? And those pills left from your son's ear infection? Throw them away immediately. You should never use someone else's prescription, not to mention an out-of-date prescription. Each person and each illness is different. Let your physician pick the appropriate antibiotic. Besides, there's another good reason to chuck the old stuff.

"Those drugs go out of date [become stale], and when they do, some of them become quite toxic. They can be harmful," says Dr. Levy.

Take all your medicine. And while we're on the subject of leftovers, what are they doing there in the first place? Most antibiotics are prescribed for a three- to seven-day period. Just because you feel better in two days doesn't mean you should stop taking your pills.

"You feel better because the majority of the bacteria have been killed, but there could be a

There are a number of steps you can take to protect yourself from resistant bacteria.

Throw away any leftover antibiotics in your medicine cabinet.

Just because you feel better in two days doesn't mean you should stop taking your pills.

minority that you have not killed," says Dr. Levy. "Once you stop the drug, they can come back and give you a second infection. The problem is that the most susceptible to antibiotics are killed in the first two days and you've left the tough guys behind. If they come back and you try the drug again, it won't be as effective."

Don't beg for antibiotics. Your physician is well acquainted with which antibiotics to prescribe for which illnesses. Antibiotics work against bacteria, not viruses. If you have a cold or flu, don't ask for antibiotics. If you do manage to find a physician who somehow justifies giving them to you, you are just adding to the problem of resistant strains of bacteria. The more antibiotics used, the worse the problem. Do the rest of us a favor and use antibiotics only when necessary.

Follow directions. This is important. Some antibiotics don't work well with certain foods. Cereals inhibit the action of tetracycline, for example. Some antibiotics must be taken with food, some on an empty stomach. And some antibiotics cause your skin to become super-sensitive to sunlight. If the doctor says to take your medicine on an empty stomach and don't go to the beach, listen and remember.

Follow directions carefully.

Watch for quick relief. If an antibiotic is going to work, you will probably see dramatic relief of your symptoms within one or two days. You won't be completely better in two days, but you should see a definite improvement. If this does not happen, let your physician know. You may be dealing with a resistant strain of bacteria, and your doctor may want to switch your medication.

Let your doctor know how you are doing.

Watch those allergies. If you have allergies, make sure your physician knows about it. Antibiotics can produce some powerful allergic reactions in some people. There is no way to know ahead of time who is going to be allergic to penicillin, for example, but if you've had a reaction to it in the past, your doctor will want to know.

Don't mix drugs. Let your physician know about any other medications you are taking, including nonprescription drugs.

Avoid raw meat. When you take antibiotics, they kill off all the bacteria you have in your gut. These bacteria provide an ecosystem that prevents infectious bacteria from moving in and causing you problems. When you take antibiotics, you are temporarily wide open.

While you should *always* avoid raw meat and poultry, be especially sure to do so when you're on antibiotics. Even a slightly resistant strain of salmonella – one that you might normally handle – can be a problem. And please, stay away from the sushi.

Yogurt can't hurt. "The bacteria in yogurt is not something that you have in your gut. When you eat yogurt, it sets up the proper environment to allow for recolonization of your intestinal tract," says Dr. Levy.

You *want* your intestinal tract recolonized with beneficial bacteria, and there is a lactobacillus in yogurt that *may* help you do that. The popular folksy advice to eat yogurt while taking antibiotics has been around for a number of years. Researchers are now looking into it. They aren't yet sure whether it really works, but downing some yogurt certainly can't hurt, says Dr. Levy. If you're going to try it, make sure the commercial yogurt you buy is made with live bacteria.

Avoid raw meats while you're on antibiotics.

Eating yogurt may introduce beneficial bacteria.

9
ANTIHISTAMINES: BLOCKING PUNCHES

Ah, spring. Ah, summer. *Ahhhh-cho-o-o-o!*

When pollen flies, even the most stalwart allergy sufferer can end up feeling like the Seven Dwarfs. Pollen hits and you go all Sneezy and Grumpy. Then you pop your antihistamine pill and suddenly you're Sleepy and Dopey. But your nose stops running and your eyes stop itching, and that makes you Happy.

Antihistamines are not, however, a fanciful bit from a fairy tale; they are a real-life wonder story. Developed in France just before World War II, antihistamines were the first drugs designed specifically to deal with the allergic reaction, says Sidney Friedlaender, M.D., clinical professor of medicine at Wayne State University School of Medicine, Detroit, and editor in chief of *Immunology and Allergy Practice*. With the possible exception of champagne, no French import has ever been received with greater enthusiasm.

Antihistamines are the medications that allergy sufferers love to hate. You can't leave home without them, but once you take them you don't *want* to leave home. You just want to go back to bed.

Antihistamines were the first drugs designed specifically to deal with the allergic reaction.

HISTAMINE PACKS A WALLOP

Antihistamines work by blocking the double-whammy punches thrown by a chemical sub-

Antihistamines work by blocking the action of histamine, a chemical your immune system produces.

77

stance that your immune system produces – histamine.

Histamine is usually bound up in granules tucked safely away inside your mast cells. Mast cells are immune cells found in your skin and the lining of your nasal passages and your gastrointestinal and respiratory tracts. The function of mast cells is not well understood, but they seem to play some kind of role in fighting viral infections. In allergic people, mast cells make trouble.

Histamine is usually bound up in granules tucked safely away inside your mast cells.

"A person who has the hereditary tendency to have this type of response will, on exposure to something that is harmless to the average person, be stimulated to develop a specific antibody, immunoglobulin E [IgE]," says Dr. Friedlaender.

Say you've inherited an allergy to ragweed pollen. The very first time you took a deep whiff of autumn air and inhaled your first ragweed pollen grains, your immune system reacted by making IgE antibodies designed specifically to latch onto ragweed pollen. You were okay that first time. But now every time you come in contact with ragweed pollen, your immune system goes bonkers.

Your first exposure to an allergen causes your immune system to make IgE antibodies that attach to mast cells.

"The IgE antibody attaches to these mast cells and these mast cells are primed. They're loaded, so to speak," says Dr. Friedlaender.

Think of all those mast cells with IgE antibodies protruding from them as a kind of minefield. Next time ragweed pollens enter your body, they bump up against those loaded mast cells and set off their chemical triggers. Your mast cells let go their load of chemicals, one of which is a nasty troublemaker known as histamine.

Subsequent exposure to the allergen causes mast cells to release histamine.

If you inject a tiny bit of synthetic histamine into your arm, it will raise a welt that looks like a mosquito bite. That's a hive. Histamines released in the nasal passages make your nose run. They also cause itchy, watery eyes and inflammation. Sound familiar?

JOIN THE FRENCH RESISTANCE

When a prizefighter throws a punch, his opponent can do one of two things if he doesn't want to take it in the chops: he can duck or he can block the punch.

When histamine throws its chemical punch, you can thank the French that there is a way to block the chemical's effect. Antihistamines won't keep your immune system from forming IgE, nor will they prevent your mast cells from unloading histamine into your body. Currently available antihistamines work by blocking the action of histamine once it's been released.

Does that mean that when you feel your allergies acting up you can just pop a pill and everything's okay? Unfortunately, nothing is ever that simple.

To get the best results from antihistamines, there are a few things you should know about.

Use antihistamines for allergy. First of all, don't treat your cold like an allergy. If what you have is a cold or flu, you might find that what you really want is a decongestant or an anti-inflammatory such as aspirin or acetaminophen (such as Tylenol).

One study conducted at Children's Hospital of Pittsburgh questioned the value of using antihistamines for relief of cold symptoms. While antihistamines helped reduce sneezing, runny noses caused by colds kept right on running. Why put up with the sometimes unpleasant side effects of antihistamines if you don't have to? Antihistamines are primarily for allergy relief.

Antihistamines are primarily for allergy relief.

Shop around. There are several different families of antihistamines available, some sold over the counter and some by prescription only.

People react to them differently. Both their effectiveness and their side effects vary from person to person. If one type of antihistamine doesn't seem to work for you or makes you too drowsy, have a go at another type.

"Read labels. If there's a question, consult a pharmacist and look for one that produces the least amount of sedation. If you've used two or three of them, you're not going to find one that works any better," says Dr. Friedlaender.

The most popular antihistamine, and the world's standard, is chlorpheniramine (Chlor-Trimeton, for example). This drug causes less drowsiness than most others and is often recommended for daytime use. Another popular one is diphenhydramine (Benadryl, for example). If diphenhydramine makes you sleepy, don't be surprised, says Dr. Friedlaender. Before it was approved for over-the-counter use as an antihistamine, it was marketed as a sleeping pill.

A few doses of an antihistamine should tell you whether or not it's going to work.

Usually only a few doses of an antihistamine will let you know whether or not it's going to work. If you try a couple of antihistamines without success, it's time to see an allergy specialist for relief.

Take your antihistamine of choice regularly and follow product directions.

Be faithful. The most effective way to take antihistamines is throughout the allergy season. Once you find your antihistamine, take it regularly to prevent symptoms from occurring in the first place.

Over-the-counter antihistamines have a long track record and are considered safe if you follow directions, says Dr. Friedlaender. Following directions means that if the box says take one tablet, you take only one tablet. You don't turn around and take two or three if the first one doesn't seem to work.

Plan ahead. If you need only occasional relief for symptoms, the trick is to remember to take antihistamines ahead of time. If you are protected from pollens in your air-conditioned house, take your antihistamines 20 to 30 minutes before going outdoors. They need time to get into your bloodstream.

A NEW GENERATION

Tired of exchanging a runny nose for that sleepy, doped-up feeling? Hang in there. A new generation of antihistamines that do not cause sleepiness is about to debut. One such product, terfenadine (Seldane) is already available by prescription only. It has tested well in its ability to provide relief. Four other new antihistamines that don't cause drowsiness – astemizole, azelastine, cetirizine, and loratidine – are already available in other countries and are currently being tested in the United States. Their effects are much longer-lasting than those of currently available antihistamines. They should be available by prescription in the near future.

Antihistamines that do not cause sleepiness are becoming available.

In the meantime, antihistamines are not the only medicines that can provide relief to seasonal allergy sufferers. Nasal steroid sprays, derived from cortisone, are available by prescription. The spray provides a localized dose of medication, and there's little or no absorption into the bloodstream.

With the number of products on the market, "it is no longer necessary for people to suffer from hay fever [allergic rhinitis]," says Dr. Friedlaender.

It is no longer necessary for people to suffer from hay fever (allergic rhinitis).

If you can't find an antihistamine that works for you, see an allergy specialist for relief, he advises.

10

ASTHMA:
BREATHING EASY

Eddie Brown was drowning. He was at the bottom of a river, struggling toward the light far above. The urge to breathe was overwhelming. The pressure in his chest was unbearable. He was suffocating. His mouth opened in a silent gasp to accept the killing water.

Eddie Brown dreamed he was drowning.

But the 42-year-old service station owner didn't drown. Instead, he broke through the sleep-dazed surface of his mind, rolled out of bed, and opened his mouth to suck in a lungful of fresh, life-giving air.

When he awakened, he was really gasping for air.

Thank God it was just a dream. Then he heard the sound. The sound was a wheeze, a rattle, the croak of a bullfrog whose bellow is muffled by the weeds at the river's edge. It was the sound of air trying to move through a pair of fluid-filled lungs gummed by mucus so thick it was like dried balls of rubber cement.

The nightmare was real. Eddie *was* drowning – drowning in the glutinous gunk produced by his own lungs.

A TWITCHY AIRWAY

Brown is one of millions of Americans who are asthmatic.

Eddie Brown is an asthmatic. He is 1 of nearly 10 million Americans who gasp their way through life because they've been cursed, as Peter S. Creticos, M.D., associate director of the Johns Hopkins Center for Asthma and Allergic

82

Diseases, explains it, with a "twitchy" airway and an "allergic potential."

What "twitchy" means, says Dr. Creticos, is that Eddie's airway – that long tube that funnels air from nostril to lung – is easily sent into spasms by various irritants (such as smoke or pollution) that usually don't affect other people. And if Eddie has an "allergic potential," he has inherited a sensitivity to specific allergens such as grasses, trees, weeds, dust, and animals.

When an allergen is inhaled through an asthmatic person's nose or mouth, explains Dr. Creticos, the protein from that allergen comes into contact with mast cells embedded in the tissue lining the airway. These mast cells have molecules of immunoglobulin E (IgE) on their surfaces. The IgE acts as a bridge between the allergen and the mast cells. And when the allergen's protein marches across this molecular bridge, the mast cells release chemical mediators (histamines, leukotrienes, prostaglandins, and enzymes) that constrict the airway, open junctures between the cells that leak fluid into the airway, and stimulate the production of a thick, sticky mucus that clogs the entire windpipe.

When an asthmatic inhales an allergen, it triggers a series of reactions that close the airways.

"The key to treatment is in controlling the chemical mediators through specific medications," says Dr. Creticos. Blocking leukotrienes, in particular, may be a major step since they are a thousand times more potent than histamines in causing bronchial constriction.

Clearly, breathing is not easy for asthmatics, says Dr. Creticos. And the problem can be particularly severe at night. A study of 7,729 British asthmatics reveals, for example, that 94 percent are awakened by nocturnal asthma once a month, while nearly 40 percent find themselves gasping for air every night. Moreover, other studies have found that most deaths due to asthma also occur at night.

The problem can be particularly severe at night.

THE IMMUNE SABOTEUR

Why do people with asthma have such a hard time getting some sleep? The asthmatic gets sabotaged by his own immune system, explains Richard Martin, M.D., an associate professor of medicine at the University of Colorado Health Sciences Center. He's being set up for an asthma attack by the natural rhythms of his own body.

Natural body rhythms can work against a person with asthma.

"These are certain circadian rhythms – body rhythms that occur in everyone every 24 hours," says Dr. Martin, who is also a staff physician at the National Jewish Center for Immunology and Respiratory Medicine in Denver. While they are perfectly natural and normal rhythms, several of them, nevertheless, can work against a person with asthma.

Histamine production reaches its peak at 4:00 A.M.

Consider the body's rhythm of producing histamine, for example. This chemical, which constricts the airway, is produced in increasing amounts during the night until it reaches a peak level at 4:00 A.M. But your body has another rhythm for producing histamine's countering agent, adrenaline. Production of this substance, which actually dilates the airway, decreases until it reaches its *lowest* level at 4:00 A.M. Other body chemicals that can help to open the airway are also lowest at night. Such syncopation in body rhythms allows histamine to tighten its grip around the asthmatic's nighttime airway. And, to make a bad situation even worse, a third circadian rhythm acts to lower body temperature. Such a drop – by itself – has been known to trigger an asthma attack.

The problem is further compounded, says Dr. Martin, by the recent discovery that your body's immune system floods the lungs with white blood cells in the middle of the night. (While other systems are at a low level, the immune system uses your sleep time to patch and repair your body.) These white blood cells release many different chemicals that can also trigger an attack. Nobody's yet figured out why they're there, which player in the immune system called them, or why they're so determined to mess up a good night's sleep.

SLEEP, SLEEP, SLEEP

Fortunately, asthma attacks – even at night – can be controlled through preventive therapy. Medications such as cromolyn, originally derived from the active ingredient of a Middle Eastern plant, can now be inhaled directly into the lungs, coating and stabilizing the airways to prevent attacks.

Furthermore, immunotherapy – injections of minute amounts of the substances you're allergic to – can trick your body's immune system into building resistance to the allergen that can trigger your attack, says Dr. Creticos.

Immunotherapy helps build resistance to the allergen that can trigger an attack.

(Note: All the immunomodulating drugs mentioned in this chapter can have serious side effects. Check with your doctor before altering your own medication or its timing.)

High doses of steroids can also be used to block asthmatic symptoms, says Dr. Martin. Exactly how steroids work is unknown, but they do block the production of some asthma-aggravating chemicals in your airway, reduce both the accumulation of fluid and mucus, and reduce some kinds of white blood cells by roughly 80 percent. Unfortunately, reducing these particular cells can also interfere with your body's ability to identify and kill at least some types of microbial invaders.

High doses of steroids can block asthmatic symptoms.

That drawback may be why many doctors seem to prefer using a drug called theophylline to both prevent and treat asthma. Theophylline controls asthma symptoms without randomly

Many doctors prefer to use a drug called theophylline to prevent and treat asthma.

shooting down masses of white cells with the scattergun approach of steroids. Instead theophylline appears to build up suppressor T-cells, the one element of your immune system that can turn off the nighttime proliferation of white cells. Theophylline increases both their numbers and activity levels. And it seems to do this without decreasing the number of helper T-cells, which your immune system needs to fight infection.

Dr. Martin says that theophylline seems to be effective in preventing nocturnal asthma only when it's taken around 7:00 P.M. in a 24-hour, timed-release preparation of Uniphyl, a theophylline drug. Other theophylline preparations, he adds, are apparently ineffective. Only the 24-hour version of Uniphyl – or, for some unknown reason, 8 hours zipped up in a tent with a good humidifier – may help the asthmatic get a good night's sleep. Even Eddie Brown.

11

CANCER:
THE NEW WAR

They come from all over the country. Some wear jeans and boots topped off with a windbreaker and a John Deere cap. Others wear wool slacks and collared sport shirts under their London Fogs. And most of them wear exhaustion. But they sit – quietly, patiently – commenting on the rain, the wind, the floods, John's cold, Bessie's fever, and whether or not Grandpa should still be driving his pickup.

When conversation drifts or pauses, they study the paintings on the stark white walls or gaze out through cathedral-size windows. And every time a man in a suit – carrying a briefcase or maybe a stethoscope – walks through the gray-carpeted reception area, they all turn their heads to watch. Where's he going? What's he doing? What's in his briefcase, his hands, his mind? Does he want me?

Their curiosity is intense because they haven't got a lot of time. Most of them are dying from advanced forms of incurable cancers and they've come here, to the Biological Therapy Institute (BTI) in Franklin, Tennessee, in hope of finding a way to stay alive.

A group of people with cancer gathers in the waiting room of a prominent cancer research institute.

A RENEGADE NCI

BTI is the clinical affiliate of Biotherapeutics, a private cancer research facility. It was set up by

Robert K. Oldham, M.D., the cancer scientist who discovered natural killer cells – those immune system commandos that target and destroy body cells that are harboring enemy invaders. Dr. Oldham then went on to set up and direct the National Cancer Institute's (NCI) Biological Response Modifiers Program in Washington, D.C.

Researchers at this institute have declared a new war on cancer.

Here, in Franklin, Dr. Oldham and 35 other leading researchers have drawn together. This elite group of scientists has set its objective as nothing less than a new war on cancer. This war, they emphasize, is one in which the most effective warriors are not stainless steel instruments but the naturally occurring components of the immune system.

It's not that the traditional therapies don't work; they just don't work for everybody.

They are waging a new war because recent federal studies report that the *old* war on cancer wasn't winning many battles. The problem, says Dr. Oldham, is not that the traditional therapies of surgery, radiation, and chemotherapy don't work. In many cases they do, and in many cases they're the appropriate treatment for a particular kind of cancer.

It's necessary to target cancer treatments directly at each individual tumor.

But not all therapies work for everyone. "What happens at the surface of a cancer cell is different from patient to patient," explains immunologist Harold Miller, Ph.D., associate scientific director at Biotherapeutics. Individual differences explain why every study ever published always has a group of patients who clearly weren't helped by the treatment. These differences also explain why it's necessary to target cancer treatments directly at each individual tumor within each individual person – rather than just saying, "Well, this kind of treatment works well a lot of the time with this kind of cancer, so let's use it." What people need, says Dr. Miller, is nothing less than their own anti-cancer prescription.

The kind of prescription that Dr. Miller is talking about often involves the immune system.

And cancer treatments involving the immune system are usually experimental, usually available only to the one out of every thousand people enrolled in federal or federally funded cancer centers, and usually only available if the center happens to be studying your particular tumor at the time you need help.

Otherwise, scientists are stuck in the lab and you're stuck at home wondering how long you've got to live.

One of the reasons Dr. Miller is at Biotherapeutics is because "I got tired of curing mice of their cancers," the immunologist says. "I wanted to see the results that we've seen in animals translated into human studies. A lot of people weren't being helped even though we knew they could be." At Biotherapeutics, he adds, anybody with advanced cancer who is in otherwise good health can literally pay for research – $2,500 to $35,000 for a custom-designed treatment specific to a particular cancer. And many of these treatments involve the immune system. Moreover, you don't have to wait for scientists to study your kind of tumor. You can start a study yourself.

At Biotherapeutics, certain people with advanced cancer can literally pay for research.

MAGIC BULLETS

The desire for a custom-made treatment explains why people are willing to give Dr. Miller and his colleagues at Biotherapeutics a chance to try out their theories. The treatment many of these people want may actually have its beginning in a narrow white room on the second floor of a nearby building.

At first the room seems like a strange place to store the magic bullets and high-tech weaponry of the immune system. There are no combination locks, flashing lights, or containers made of a new alloy. No test tubes, Bunsen burners,

These specialized treatments involve the magic bullets and high-tech weaponry of the immune system.

This anti-cancer weaponry includes lymphokines, MAbs, and TDAC.

flasks, or beakers connected by miles of plastic tubing and years of study. Those are across the hall, tended by white-coated technicians and the scientists who work with them.

In this small room there aren't any people – just 12 waist-high containers that look like heavy-duty trash cans from Sears. Although it doesn't look like the frontier of immunology, it is. And the words casually scrawled in black felt-tip across each container reveal the lethal magic within. "Lymphokines," "MAbs," "TDAC," and one marked – perhaps more carefully – "tumors."

The contents of these trash cans are unlike anything else in the world.

Lymphokines serve as chemical messengers for the immune system.

Lymphokines, for example, are chemical messengers that carry instructions from one part of your immune system to another. Two of them, interleukin-1 (IL-1) and interleukin-2 (IL-2), were accidentally discovered by two Yale University researchers who cultured macrophages in a broth and then threw them out. When they later added T-cells to the same broth, the researchers were surprised to discover that the T-cells multiplied. Somehow, something in the broth, something left over from the macrophages, had turbocharged the T-cells.

The "something," scientists later discovered, was interleukin, a naturally occurring chemical secreted by the macrophages. Did this discovery indicate that it was possible to rev up the immune system's components to fight diseases such as cancer? And was interleukin the component that could do it?

Maybe. But as scientists watched new batches of T-cells stimulated by interleukin grow in the lab, they began to realize that mature T-cells secreted several substances of their own. One is IL-2, the mysterious turbocharger that apparently activated the T-cells. Moreover, it's IL-2, scientists say, that acts directly on the T-cells to produce the killer cells capable of annihilating cancer.

PROGRAMMING YOUR IMMUNE SYSTEM TO KILL

Can Interleukin-2, then, program your immune system to kill cancer? Yes. But which kind of cancer, and when and how it works, has remained something of a mystery.

Further research into IL-2 was at first slow because only minute amounts were available for scientists to experiment with. Since the development of genetic engineering techniques, however, IL-2 has been pouring into both labs and clinics and scientists have been experimenting with amounts, concentrations, combinations, schedules, and administration.

The result of this experimentation is an explosion of information. Investigators at the NCI, for example, have discovered that high doses of IL-2 apparently can cause the regression of some types of cancer, particularly melanoma.

NCI investigators have also discovered that if they remove some white blood cells from cancer patients, incubate them with IL-2 in the lab, then shoot the cells – now renamed lymphokine activated killer (LAK) cells – back into patients with another dose of IL-2, they can shrink the patients' cancers in *half*.

Further study at the NCI has confirmed that this treatment – called adoptive immunotherapy – can reduce or occasionally eliminate even advanced, rapidly spreading cancer in just over a third of the patients who receive it. In a study of 106 patients, investigators found it was particularly effective in those with kidney cancer and melanoma.

Now, reducing a cancerous tumor by a third or even a half may not sound like a wildly successful treatment. And what good does it do to "reduce" cancer? "It reduces the tumor burden on your immune system," explains Ronald B. Herberman, M.D., a former director of NCI's Biological Response Modifiers Program who is

Genetic engineering techniques have made more Interleukin-2 available for study.

LAK cells, made with IL-2, can shrink patients' cancers in *half*.

This treatment can reduce or occasionally eliminate even advanced, rapidly spreading cancer.

now director of the Pittsburgh Cancer Institute. If a treatment can lighten that load, he says, "your immune system will have a good chance to eliminate the residual cancer" on its own.

Tragically, several people died in the NCI studies, either because of infection from contaminated cells or cultures or because they were simply too ill to weather the grueling side effects of Interleukin-2. Naturally occurring or not, extra IL-2 can affect both heart and lung function. In one study of IL-2 alone, for example, eight out of ten patients received a portion of their treatment in the research facility's intensive care unit.

Because of these events, doctors seemed to give up hope that IL-2 could ever be used, except in the lab. Editorials in major American medical journals condemned the investigators and seemed to imply that they should allow cancer patients to die in peace.

Research at Biotherapeutics has apparently overcome the major side effects.

The scientists at Biotherapeutics, however, weren't listening. Their work continued unabated, and now they apparently have solved the problems behind these treatment-related deaths. To keep the LAK cells from being contaminated by any infectious agents, lab director John Yannelli, Ph.D., invented a closed laboratory system. And to make the treatment easier on cancer patients, medical director William H. West, M.D., proceeded to give LAK cells back to the patient in a steady infusion over a five-day period rather than as a single shot every 8 hours. Thus, Biotherapeutics has apparently overcome the major side effects.

THE LATEST WRINKLE

Researchers incubate a piece of the patient's tumor with IL-2 to create TDAC cells.

Adoptive immunotherapy, however, is still evolving. The latest wrinkle, says Dr. Miller, is to take a slice of the patient's tumor – not just his white cells, but a piece of the tumor itself – and incubate it in the lab with IL-2. After several days small armies of tumor-derived activated cells (TDAC) will appear and eradicate the tumor. When nothing is left but TDAC, doctors can take that substance, mix it with another round of IL-2, and give it back to the person that the tumor came from. Usually an immunosuppressant drug is given before the cells are returned so the person's suppressor T-cells are less likely to sabotage the TDAC attack.

How effective is TDAC? The NCI, which calls the substance tumor infiltrating lymphocytes, reports that it seems to be between 50 and 100 times more potent than LAK cell immunotherapy. It is, after all, a killer specifically made to attack a particular tumor rather than just boosting the immune system in general, as does LAK.

Studies with people are now in progress, but in the meantime, laboratory studies indicate that scientists can expect astounding results. With the combination of an immunosuppressant drug, TDAC and IL-2, for example, all the colon cancers – that's 100 percent – that had spread to the liver in laboratory mice were cured. Fifty percent of the lung cancers were also cured, and the mice, which would normally have survived 17 or 18 days without treatment, lived for more than 100.

Scientists can expect astounding results with the combination of immunosuppressant drugs, TDAC, and IL-2.

But that's still not good enough for Dr. Miller. "What we want to do now, is to load the TDAC cells with antibodies and – Wham! – kill the tumor," he says. "This will assure an ongoing assault until live tumor cells weaken and die."

What Dr. Miller refers to is growing an army of killer cells in the lab and loading them onto a guided missile called a monoclonal antibody (MAb), which is then targeted at the cancer tumor. MAb is usually made by injecting a cancer patient's tumor cells into a mouse, killing the mouse, and harvesting the B-cells that are produced in response to the tumors. A single cell is then wedded to a kind of deactivated myeloma cancer cell and allowed to proliferate. The off-

Researchers now want to load TDAC cells onto monoclonal antibodies.

spring of this unholy alliance is a cell-producing antibody called a monoclonal because it has been cloned *(clonal)* from a single *(mono)* B-cell.

MAbs can be delivered to the tumor with chemicals and radioactive particles.

On occasion, MAbs can kill cancer cells themselves by activating the complement system. More often, they can be laden with a variety of toxins, drugs, chemicals, or radioactive isotopes and delivered to the tumor, says Dr. Miller. Molecules of diphtheria toxin, for example, can be loaded onto the MAb and sent to a tumor, where they will literally penetrate the tumor with diphtheria and poison it. Or a radioactive particle can be loaded onto the MAb and sent to a tumor where it will destroy the cancer cell with localized radiation.

MAb delivery is tricky—the MAb is easily sidetracked.

But MAb delivery is tricky. The MAb and its toxic warhead are injected into the bloodstream, where they're supposed to circulate to the tumor. In reality, says Dr. Miller, the MAb is easily sidetracked. Minute particles of tumor circulating in your blood can effectively act as a decoy and lure the MAb away from its target. Or the MAbs can get trapped in an organ such as the lungs or liver. Or, since they're generally made from a mouse's B-cell, your immune system can think there's a mouse running around in your arteries and try to shoot it down with its own antirodent defense system.

Biotherapeutics scientists think they can overcome some of the MAb's inherent problems.

That's why scientists at Biotherapeutics like to custom-tailor a MAb to your particular tumor. It takes nine months in the lab, but by modifying the MAb-making process to use human rather than mouse cells, Biotherapeutics scientists think they can overcome some of the MAb's inherent problems. Not only is a custom-tailored MAb more likely to fit – and, thus, destroy – your tumor target, says Dr. Miller, but it's less likely to trigger your antirodent defenses as well.

Many people with cancer don't have time to wait around for a custom job, however, so Biotherapeutics maintains a library of hundreds of "off the rack" MAbs that it shares with research institutes across the country. The library MAbs don't always bind quite as well to each individual's tumor as the custom-tailored ones, says Dr. Miller, so they're probably not as effective. But if you've got a fast-growing tumor, they're clearly very powerful backups that are worth a shot.

"LOBSTERS" ON THE FRONTIER

How else can the immune system and its components be manipulated to treat cancer? Interferon, a substance secreted by mature T-cells in response to viral infections, has been found to kill tumor cells in several cancers, particularly hairy cell leukemia (it can reduce 90 percent of it); Kaposi's sarcoma (30 percent); non-Hodgkin's lymphomas; chronic myelogenous leukemia; and kidney, skin, and bladder cancers. It may affect even more cancers, scientists say, but so far they've only studied 3 of its estimated 20 faces.

And thymosin, a powerful hormone secreted by the thymus, has also been shown to affect the immune system's response to tumors. Laboratory studies indicate that it can zip up suppressed or depressed T-cells, although this effect has not yet been demonstrated in people.

At Biotherapeutics, however, the major thrust of research seems to be directed toward developing more specific, more toxic warheads and loading them onto MAbs.

In fact, says Tim O'Connor, Ph.D., the associate scientific director who was formerly director of biomedical research at the prestigious Roswell Park Memorial Institute, one of the things he'd most like to do is hook a substance that attracts macrophages onto the tail of the lobster-shaped MAbs. The "lobster claws" would clamp onto the tumor and a macrophage – which actually came to eat the "lobster tail" – would end up eating the tumor as well, because tumor and tail are attached. This approach – antibody de-

Interferon and thymosin are also being used to treat cancers.

pendent cellular cytolysis – works well in the test tube, says Dr. O'Connor, but he wants to know more about how it can work in people.

Dr. O'Connor wants to investigate ways to reprogram the immune system during various stages of its battle with cancer.

He also wants to look into more ways to reprogram the immune system during various stages of its battle with cancer. Look at how the immune system fights the schistosoma parasite in tropical countries, he suggests. The schistosomas enter your body from snails' worm larvae as you walk through infested waters or rice paddies. They then travel in your bloodstream to the liver, gut, or bladder, where they mate and produce millions of eggs.

But people live quite a while with this disease, says Dr. O'Connor. And the reason is that at different stages of the infestation, their immune system shifts gears and uses different responses to keep it in check.

The idea is to issue a new set of instructions telling the immune system how to attack in new ways.

Why can't scientists use this metaphor in cancer therapy? asks Dr. O'Connor. If a cancer that was originally "cured" with chemotherapy recurs, for example, chemotherapy frequently won't work a second time. So the idea – borrowed from the schistosoma invader – is to issue a new set of instructions to your immune system that tells it how to attack in new ways. Instead of curing cancer, you may simply learn how to manipulate your immune system to keep it in check.

That's why the research into the possibility that lymphokines can continuously reprogram your immune system is so important, says Dr. O'Connor. Imagine that research into lymphokines is like playing pool. At first it looks easy – all you have to do is break the rack and knock a few balls into the side pocket. But what if every time a ball drops into the pocket, five more appear on the table? The incessant development of new discoveries explains why research into the immune system is so time consuming, says Dr. O'Connor. Every time you figure out how one substance affects a particular component, you realize that the component you're studying affects another and another and another. Since scientists suspect there are more than 100 lymphokines issuing orders to your immune system, it'll probably take them years to even *find* the eight ball, much less figure out how to sink it.

GIVING YOUR IMMUNE SYSTEM A BOOST

The difficulty in developing cancer treatments is why it's so important to prevent cancer in the first place. How? By keeping your immune system tuned to maximum efficiency.

It's important to prevent cancer in the first place.

Your immune system is constantly on guard against any cancer invasion, explains the Pittsburgh Cancer Institute's Dr. Herberman. A group of cancer cells begins to grow, they're detected by your immune system, and certain killer cells are deployed to zap the evolving tumor before you knew it was there. The system, however, is not perfect. "The ability of your immune system to control cancer is somewhat limited," says Dr. Herberman. "If there's an extensive amount, it can overwhelm your defenses."

To keep your defenses on the alert, he advises, you need to eat a well-balanced diet that pays particular attention to vitamins B and C, and limit your exposure to cancer-causing agents such as cigarette smoke and sunlight.

Keep your immune system's cancer defenses on the alert.

And because inadequate amounts of sleep, exercise, and play are also thought to suppress your immune system, some doctors suggest you avoid late nights, get a moderate amount of exercise, and make sure you take time to laugh.

Think that's funny, do you? Good. Keep laughing. Because keeping your T-cells in stitches also builds your immune system. And that may be the only difference between you and someone waiting for a cancer treatment in Franklin, Tennessee.

12

COLDS: BEYOND CHICKEN SOUP

Oh, no. Not again. You've got 437 errands to run. The cat needs to go to the vet. Your mother has to be dropped at the eye doctor's. And your son is probably waiting – covered with mud and dripping with sweat – for you to pick him up at soccer.

But instead of rushing out the door to meet the expectations of a demanding world, you sit in your chair, exhausted. Your nose is stuffy, your throat feels scratchy, and you have the I'm-going-to-sneeze prickles.

Yes, you've got a cold. And you can, of course, ignore it. Or you can treat it with lots of fluids, a few days in bed, and a half-dozen decongestants, and it will disappear in seven days. Either way you're in for a miserable week. How can a lousy little virus make you feel so rotten?

A TWINKLE OF GENETIC MATERIAL

Actually, it's not the virus that makes you feel so bad, it's you, says David Proud, Ph.D., a research immunologist at Johns Hopkins University School of Medicine.

Your cold causes the release of inflammatory chemicals in your nose called kinins.

Your cold – usually sparked by a minute twinkle of genetic material called a rhinovirus – triggers a process that results in the release of inflammatory chemicals in your nose called kinins, explains Dr. Proud. The kinins, which are made by your body in response to the invading virus, apparently cause blood vessels in the nose to swell and leak. The swelling obstructs your nose, the leak causes it to run, and when the kinins drip down the back of your throat, they keep producing the pain that makes you feel like you're swallowing a cactus.

Fortunately, says Dr. Proud, your nose doesn't seem to have the pain receptors that are sensitive to kinin. Otherwise you'd probably be trying to stick the same anesthetic lozenges up your nose as down your throat.

TURNING OFF THE WATERWORKS

A theory of the way kinins work, proposed by Dr. Proud and his colleagues, has changed forever the way we handle colds. For years, Dr. Proud explains, scientists thought that histamines – chemicals secreted by your immune system in response to an allergy – were not only responsible for the runny eyes and noses of pollen season but for the waterworks display during a cold. So doctors usually prescribed antihistamines – Benadryl and Chlor-Trimeton, for example – to relieve cold symptoms.

But antihistamines never subdue a cold as effectively as they snuff out an allergy attack. And now, of course, we know why. Since histamines don't trigger the symptoms, antihistamines can't stop them. Fortunately, anti*kinins* should.

"We've shown that kinins are present when symptoms are present, that they're absent when symptoms are absent, that when you introduce them to the relevant site, they induce the relevant symptoms," says Dr. Proud. "But the third, big, crucial point [in drug research] is that you have to be able to go in there and interfere with their actions and show that antikinins affect

A theory of the way kinins work has changed forever the way we handle colds.

Researchers have shown that kinins are present when such symptoms are present.

symptoms. And that's what we're going to try to do now."

A MICROGRAM OF PREVENTION

While Dr. Proud and his colleagues at Johns Hopkins are trying to relieve your cold symptoms, however, Frederick Hayden, M.D., a viral researcher at the University of Virginia Medical School, is trying to figure out how to prevent your cold to begin with. And – to some extent – he actually seems to have succeeded.

Dr. Hayden and his colleagues have been studying alpha interferon, a synthetic protein molecule that calls your immune system's heavy artillery – the natural killer cells – into action. In one study they conducted, for example, 60 families from the Charlottesville area demonstrated that alpha interferon prevented colds in 90 percent of the family members who were exposed to a cold virus.

The families, which included two adults between the ages of 18 and 75 and two children between the ages of 2 and 17, were split into two groups. One group was given a metered-dose nasal spray of interferon, while the other was given a nasal spray with a fake – and ineffective – solution. Neither group knew which spray was real and which was fake. Both groups were told that, if one member of the family came down with a cold, the other members were to give themselves two squirts of "interferon" once each morning for the next seven days. They also had to call the University of Virginia so that a staff member could come and collect a nasal sample for laboratory analysis.

After eight months, Dr. Hayden and his colleagues tabulated the results: among people exposed to laboratory-documented colds – roughly a quarter of the study's participants – illness developed in 12 of 34 people who were

Researchers are studying a substance that calls your immune system's heavy artillery into action.

They are testing interferon nasal spray.

given the fake solution, but in only 2 of the 27 given interferon.

Clearly, interferon prevents colds. But the study also revealed that by giving interferon in this particular dose and in this particular way, the researchers had apparently found a way to overcome the side effects of industrial-strength interferon. Even though interferon is naturally produced in the body, the artifically high doses used for prolonged periods had produced nasal irritation and blood-tinged mucus in previous studies. When used only on the two-squirts-a-day-for-one-week basis of Dr. Hayden's study, the side effects – predominantly inflammation – occurred in only three people.

> Interferon prevents colds, but there are problems with side effects.

"The way we expect people to use this," says Dr. Hayden, "is as *we* used it in the study – to protect the family when one of its members gets a cold. Hopefully, it will be available in the near future."

VIRAL "BIRTH CONTROL"

There's at least one immunological strategy that scientists are using to prevent colds. One molecular virologist, working with a top pharmaceutical company, has developed it.

> One researcher is working to stop the action of the cold virus in the nose.

Realizing that people are always playing with their faces, he came up with a good, simple idea. If your nose is the only place a cold virus can effectively enter your body, that's where a cold can be stopped. Tissue in your nose has projections, shaped like lightning rods, that attract the cold virus the way, well, the way a lightning rod attracts lightning. A cold virus, in return, has a deep, narrow crevice – some call it a canyon – into which the projection fits. And when the two meet – when the projection tickles the genetic material at the bottom of the crevice – the virus reproduces itself – 100 times!

He is developing a type of viral "birth control."

Your immune system can't get to the bottom of the crevice and neutralize the virus. So what's needed is something akin to birth control for the virus. In this case the prophylactic is a monoclonal antibody that fits over the projections in your nose like a sheath, blocking any contact between projections and virus and preventing the production of any offspring. And this method of "birth control" is 100 percent effective in the laboratory.

With no one to make love to, the virus gets washed down your throat and into your stomach, where the natural acidity of your gastrointestinal tract destroys it. You never even get a sniffle.

WORKING OUT THE BUGS

Diagnostic kits may someday help your doctor treat your cold.

Monoclonal antibodies to prevent your cold won't hit the drugstore for quite a while, experts say. But the approach that they're using is so customized to a particular type of virus that your doctor – or you, since it will probably be available over the counter – would have to have some kind of diagnostic kit where you could take a mucus sample, rub it on a strip and maybe one little circle would turn red. Each circle would indicate a different group of viruses, of course, and each group would probably have a different monoclonal-based drug to treat it.

These diagnostic kits also are in the future. In the meantime, the monoclonal antibody currently under the microscope is partially made from mouse cells. Unfortunately, there's always the danger – as with monoclonals that are used in cancer therapy – that your body's immune system will think you've got mice running around in your arteries and launch an all-out attack.

If you have cancer, you might want to take that risk. But, if you have a cold, the cure could be worse than the disease. Since the foreign antibody would be used each time you get a cold, a person might develop a hyperimmune response to it – a response similar to an allergic reaction. The mild symptoms of a virus are far preferable to those of an immune system hunting rodents. Even if you do have 437 errands.

COLD COMFORT

While we're waiting for these developments to appear on our drugstore shelves, however, here are a few tips to help you make it through your cold:

Drink a glass of water or juice every 2 or 3 hours. It'll flush the virus out of your system and replace any fluids that you've lost. A runny nose – especially if combined with a mild fever – can put you on the uncomfortable road to dehydration.

Try gargling with apple cider vinegar mixed with honey if your throat is a little sore. The recipe, which originated in New England, is 1 or 2 teaspoons of honey with 1 or 2 teaspoons of apple cider vinegar and water. You can also suck on ice chips or throat lozenges that contain menthol. Both have that ahhhhh-that's-better effect.

Use a nasal decongestant to clear your stuffy nose. Local decongestants are more powerful than oral ones, doctors say, and spray decongestants – which penetrate even your sinuses – are better than nose drops. The best way to use a decongestant is to spray each nostril once, wait 5 minutes, then spray a second time. The first shot will shrink swollen membranes in your nose, the second will clear your sinuses. If you want to avoid the rebound effect – a stuffiness that's caused by using the spray so long it starts to cause the problem it's supposed to cure – buy a mild spray such as 0.25% percent Neo-Synephrine. You can use it for up to a month without any problem.

If you prefer oral decongestants, use pseudoephedrine (Sudafed, for example) and phenyl-

There are a number of ways to help you make it through your cold.

Drink fluids and try gargling if your throat is a little sore.

Use decongestants to clear stuffiness.

propanolamine (like Unitrol). They're both available over the counter at your local pharmacy.

Don't forget Mom's chicken soup. Actually, any hot, steamy beverage will liquify secretions and relieve congestion. But a mug of hot chicken soup with as many mashed cloves of garlic as friends, lovers, and neighbors will tolerate is claimed – by some doctors at least – to be the best.

Get plenty of rest.

Take it easy. The effort required to fight cold germs – especially during the first few days – is the equivalent of hard physical labor. While you don't have to hit the sack at the onset of a cold, you should putter rather than push yourself. Limiting activities during a cold's early stages also can reduce the chances that you'll spread your cold around. Colds are most contagious shortly after they strike.

Stay warm and don't smoke.

Keep bundled up. To combat the chills that can accompany a cold, give your body's defenses the advantage of keeping as comfortably toasty as possible.

Do not smoke. Especially not now. Smoking can further irritate an already agonized respiratory tract as well as depress the body's levels of vitamin C – a vitamin intimately connected with maintaining your body's immune system. What's more, it can paralyze structures in the lungs – the cilia – needed to keep breathing passages as free as possible of mucus.

Cough. A "productive" cough helps your body clear the gunk out of your airway. Don't try to suppress it. Unless you have asthma or chronic bronchitis, *dry* coughs should be soothed with a hot shower, hard candy, a throat lozenge, or a dose of dextromethorphan, an over-the-counter cough remedy available under 50 different brand names. Of course, any cough that lasts longer than a few days should be evaluated by your doctor.

13

CUTS, BURNS, AND BRUISES: GUARDING THE BORDER

Skin: the initial frontier. The place where you end and the sky begins. The carefully guarded borderland between your body and the rest of the world.

Skin is your protective barrier. When it is breached, you are in trouble. This is not intended to make you paranoid, but the great, wide world crawls with things that long to get under your skin. Bacteria, viruses, fungi, and parasites are just like you in the sense that they need warmth, shelter, and nourishment. Your body provides those things in abundance for any microbe lucky enough to get through your protective outer skin and evade your immune system's defenses.

Skin serves as your protective barrier against germs.

Microbes know a good thing when they see it. To you, a cut or a burn is a violation of your body. To them, those breaches in your skin look like the doorway to a microbe cafeteria.

Here's how to assist your immune system's border patrol and help stop alien invaders before they turn into an infection.

You can help your immune system prevent infection.

UNKIND CUTS

The unkindest cut of all is the cut that becomes infected. That's why cleaning a cut and keeping it clean while it heals are absolutely vital. But what to use?

Keeping a cut clean while it heals is vital.

Contrary to the loving treatment you received at mother's knee as a child, the old regimen of soap and water followed by a generous swabbing of Mercurochrome might not be the best idea.

Many soaps, it turns out, are highly irritating to fresh wounds, according to Patricia Mertz, research associate professor of dermatology at the University of Miami School of Medicine. Mertz works with a team of physicians and researchers who study the way wounds heal. They evaluate the effectiveness of various treatments both on patients in a clinical setting and on human volunteers in the laboratory. What they have discovered may surprise you.

Strong soaps clean the wound all right, says Mertz, but they also kill the delicate new tissues forming as a part of the healing process. That's not good, because the longer it takes a cut to heal, the longer you leave the door open to infection. A wash with *mild* soap and water is okay, but there are better alternatives.

Mercurochrome, the red stuff you probably had your knees painted with as a child, is not a good idea either. Also known as tincture of Merthiolate, the active ingredient in this popular antiseptic can cause an allergic reaction – or, in the allergy-prone, even create new allergies to related substances.

Superficial cuts should not be treated with strong soaps and antiseptics.

"Superficial cuts should not be treated aggressively. They shouldn't be treated with strong soaps and antiseptics," says Mertz. "Hydrogen peroxide is probably a better way to go. Hydrogen peroxide will remove the foreign material without harming the tissue."

Nor should you wrap a cut or wound with dry gauze.

"Newly forming epidermis grows into the gauze and as you remove it – you can probably remember doing this as a child – it hurts," warns Mertz. "It hurts because you're removing not only the crust but also the newly formed tissue that's supposed to protect you from infection.

"There is some evidence that the best way to reduce scarring is to use a dressing that keeps the healing tissue moist. And some of the antibiotic ointments speed wound healing for this same reason. They decrease the amount of crust that forms. The tissue stays moist, and this allows healing to take place more rapidly."

There are new types of gauze on the market as well as numerous types of dressings that keep cuts moist while they heal. Ask your pharmacist about them. Even bandages that have a plastic film help keep cuts moist, Mertz advises.

"As a topical product, I would suggest polymyxin B sulfate ointment," she says.

For people who can tolerate it, antibiotic cream containing neomycin is excellent, says Mertz, "but dermatologists don't like to suggest it because there's a certain portion of the population that is allergic to neomycin. It might make your cut worse if you have an allergy to it."

In general, you should watch for allergic reactions to any topical product that you use. If a rash develops, discontinue use immediately.

If you receive a deep puncture wound rather than a cut, you are especially at risk for infection. Punctures from things like rusty nails inject dirt deep beneath the skin and rarely bleed enough to clean it out. You need to see a physician. You may need antibiotics and a tetanus shot if your booster is not up to date.

> **The best way to reduce scarring is to use a dressing that keeps the healing tissue moist.**

> **Antibiotic creams containing neomycin are excellent.**

> **Tetanus shots may be required for puncture wounds.**

BEASTLY BURNS

If cuts provide an entryway for microbes, burns are a veritable highway. Burn away the top layer of skin, and you are wide open for infection.

Okay, you've been burned. What do you do now?

Serious burns leave you open for infection and require professional help.

If it doesn't hurt, and you can see that you've been burned – the skin has turned white – you've got a third-degree burn. This means that the entire thickness of skin has been destroyed. Don't try to treat this type of burn yourself. Seek professional help.

You can treat a *small* second-degree burn yourself.

A partial thickness burn, or second-degree burn, hurts. There's blistering, and the skin is moist and weepy-looking. You can treat a *small* second-degree burn yourself, provided it covers an area no greater in size than the palm of the victim's hand.

First-degree burns are superficial burns that do not blister. The skin is red and dry but still intact. Most sunburns fall into this category.

The first thing to do following a minor burn is to apply cold water, advises Mertz. Dip the affected part in cold water, run cold water over it, or apply a cloth that has been soaked in cold water. The cold water helps reduce pain and inflammation.

If you raise a blister, gently dry it with sterile gauze or a clean cloth, then cover it. Don't try to open the blister. The skin of the blister, if it remains intact, will help prevent infection.

BOTHERSOME BRUISES

Bruises are caused by bleeding into the tissues beneath the skin.

The various blues and greens of bruises are caused by bleeding into the tissues beneath the skin. It is blue rather than red because that's the color of blood that has not been exposed to oxygen. You don't have to worry about infection, but bruises do still challenge your immune system. Macrophages, cells that serve as a clean-up crew for your immune system, have to physically carry off blood that leaks out under your skin.

Treat bruises with ice or cold water to reduce swelling.

14

DIABETES:
THE SWEET NEWS

More than just a sweet dream, the possibility of a cure for diabetes shimmers on the horizon. The hoped-for cure is still just beyond grasp, but it is coming ever closer.

A cure for diabetes is a growing possibility.

One of the leading causes of death in America, the dread disease may soon succumb to the big guns of medical science. And the key to both the cause and the cure of the most serious form of that disease seems to lie in the immune system.

Diabetes is a disease that interferes with your body's fuel-delivery system. Sugar serves as your energy source. To keep your living motor running, the sweet fuel that drives your body has to reach every single cell. You require a steady supply.

Diabetes interferes with your body's energy supply—sugar.

We're not talking table sugar here. Your digestive system breaks down the food that you eat into a number of things that your body needs, including simple sugars. Even a slice of bread is turned into sugars for your body to run on. But with diabetes, the fuel that the body needs can't get where it needs to go.

For a quick picture of how this works, consider your family car for a moment. You can pump super octane gasoline into the fuel tank, but if the fuel injector is on the fritz or the fuel filter is plugged, forget it. The engine may ping, stall, or even . . . you'll pardon the expression . . . die.

So what does all this have to do with your immune system?

IMMUNE SYSTEM REBELLION

Your body needs insulin to carry sugar to your cells.

Your body relies on some fairly complicated chemistry to carry the sugars extracted from your food to your cells. It needs insulin, produced in your pancreas, to do the job.

The more serious form of diabetes is now known to be *autoimmune*.

The more serious form of diabetes, the kind of diabetes that children often get, is now known to be *autoimmune,* according to George Eisenbarth, M.D., Ph.D., associate professor of medicine at Harvard Medical School and chief of the Section of Immunology at Joslin Diabetes Center. Scientists have come to that understanding only within the last 15 years, and it will make all the difference in the world in terms of future treatment, says Dr. Eisenbarth.

Autoimmune disease is what happens when the immune system makes a mistake. The immune system gets confused and, for reasons that medical science does not entirely understand, it turns around and attacks parts of the body. To get a picture of autoimmunity, imagine what happens in a war when the artillery makes a mistake and lobs shells on its own soldiers.

The immune system attacks the cells in the pancreas that produce insulin.

There are two types of diabetes. In insulin-dependent (Type I) diabetes, the disease that usually strikes children, the immune system attacks the cells in the pancreas that produce insulin and knocks them out of commission. No insulin-producing cells means no insulin. And no insulin means the sugar that the digestive system releases into the bloodstream can't get where it's supposed to go. Instead of being fed to the body as sweet living energy, the sugar bounces around in the blood vessels doing damage.

And when muscle cells can't burn sugar, they have to consume something else for their energy. So they start to burn fat instead, and the resulting fatty acid residues leave deposits in the arteries. That's why diabetics are more likely to develop hardening of the arteries and heart disease.

Non-insulin-dependent (Type II) diabetes, on the other hand, is not an autoimmune disease. Also known as adult-onset diabetes, it's the more common form of the disease.

In non-insulin-dependent diabetes, the pancreas continues to produce insulin. But the body's cells have a hard time receiving the sugar that is being delivered to them. Although still a very serious disease, non-insulin-dependent diabetes can be controlled and even prevented through diet, weight control, and exercise.

In non-insulin-dependent diabetes, the pancreas continues to produce insulin.

A GROWING MENACE

The American Diabetes Association estimates that 11 million Americans have diabetes, and of that number, only 7 million have been diagnosed. Approximately 10 to 15 percent of the people who have the disease have the insulin-dependent type.

The incidence of insulin-dependent diabetes is rising alarmingly. It has apparently tripled in the last 50 years, according to Dr. Eisenbarth. And researchers don't yet know why.

The incidence of insulin-dependent diabetes has tripled in the last 50 years.

In animals, diet has an impact on the development (or nondevelopment) of the disease. And so do certain viruses. Researchers just don't know whether the growing incidence of the disease is due to dietary changes, environmental changes, genetic mutation, or something else.

Researchers don't know what is causing the increase.

"It could be some virus that we catch that changes the immune system. In man, we only know of one such environmental factor. That's congenital rubella. Rubella infection affects the fetus's developing immune system, and it is changed for life," says Dr. Eisenbarth.

EARLY DETECTION NOW POSSIBLE

Early diagnosis is vital.

Because insulin-dependent diabetes is so damaging, the earlier that it is diagnosed and treated, the better. Immune system monitoring has made early detection possible. That is good news for families that suffer from a high rate of diabetes. They will soon be able to monitor their children and spot the development of the disease years before it manifests itself.

Insulin-dependent diabetes develops in six stages, says Dr. Eisenbarth.

Something triggers the disease in genetically susceptible people.

First, a genetic predisposition must be present. Diabetes runs in families. People with immediate relatives who have diabetes are much more likely to develop the disease. Second, there is some sort of trigger that sets off the disease. Researchers don't yet have a handle on what that trigger might be. It could be dietary or something in the environment, like a virus.

In the final stages of diabetes, all the insulin-producing cells are destroyed.

Once the disease is triggered, the immune system takes an abnormal turn that targets pancreas cells for destruction. That is stage three. At stage four, insulin production falls off. At stage five, enough of the insulin-producing pancreas cells have been killed off to create problems. That is when people become aware that they have the disease. At this point they may have had the disease for years. A good deal of damage has already been done without them even being aware of it. And at stage six, all the insulin-producing cells have been destroyed.

The importance of recognizing all these stages in the development of diabetes is that researchers can now see the disease coming well before it begins to do serious damage. Auto-antibodies – antibodies that the immune system makes against the body's own insulin-producing cells – and other immune system products show up in the blood, revealing that the destructive process of the disease is under way.

Although these detection procedures are still in the testing stages, it is already possible to screen children who are at risk for the disease and catch the disease early. Undiagnosed diabetes can kill, so that's important.

It is now possible to diagnose the disease sooner.

These screening tests have not yet been standardized, so you cannot yet go to your physician and ask for them. But researchers all over the world are working on them, and the tests should soon be widely available, according to Dr. Eisenbarth.

PREVENTION RESEARCH HOLDS HOPE

"The other major question is if you know someone's developing diabetes, what will you do about it? That also is in the realm of clinical research right now," says Dr. Eisenbarth.

Researchers are looking into ways to treat and prevent diabetes.

Dr. Eisenbarth investigated dietary factors that might prevent the disease, so far without much success. Nicotinamide, a form of B vitamin, prevents diabetes in one type of diabetes-prone mice. His research showed, unfortunately, that it does not have the same effect in humans.

Epidemiologists, scientists who study the relationship of populations and disease distributions, are also looking for dietary answers to diabetes. Maybe someday they'll be able to tell us what to eat, and what not to eat, to keep from getting the disease.

Meanwhile, the most promising research into treatments for insulin-dependent diabetes involves drugs that affect the immune system.

Drugs that affect the immune system hold some promise.

In tests conducted in Paris and elsewhere, children with insulin-dependent diabetes were treated with cyclosporine, a drug that suppresses the immune system. Test results were promising. Cyclosporine is the drug that is given to organ transplant patients to keep their immune systems from rejecting the transplanted organs. In the Paris study, more than half of the children given the drug were able to discontinue insulin shots four months after beginning the drug treatment.

Cyclosporine has serious side effects.

Cyclosporine is no magic bullet, however. The drug works by suppressing the immune system, which does, after all, protect the body from infection. The drug also produces some serious side effects.

"The major problem is kidney toxicity," says Dr. Eisenbarth. "If it weren't for that, it would probably be used right now for preventing diabetes, despite the risk of moderate immune suppression. But a number of trials are trying to get around the problem."

Much of the research work aimed at controlling diabetes looks promising and may yield concrete results within the next few years. That is sweet news for anyone who suffers from the sugar disease.

PREVENTING TYPE II DIABETES

One form of diabetes can be controlled through diet and exercise.

The news is even sweeter for adults who have developed non-insulin-dependent diabetes. You can control this form of diabetes and even prevent it, through diet and exercise.

"At least 90 percent of the cases of non-insulin-dependent diabetes could be prevented if people would get to their ideal weight and stay there," says John Davidson, M.D., Ph.D, director of the diabetes clinic at Emory University's Grady Memorial Hospital.

People with this form of diabetes are more susceptible to infection.

Although non-insulin-dependent diabetes is not an autoimmune disease, it can have a major impact on the immune system. People with this form of diabetes are more susceptible to infection if the disease is not controlled.

"If the blood sugar is high, you develop a condition that makes you more susceptible to candida, staphylococcus, and all the other infectious agents. And people don't respond as well to treatment as they would if their blood sugar were normal," says Dr. Davidson.

"For the vast majority of the non-insulin-dependent, we know the cause of their diabetes, which is being overweight, and we've got the cure.

"The only thing we've got to do is convince the physicians who are dealing with them to treat them with diet and get them to lose weight."

DON'T BECOME A STATISTIC

The number of Americans who have non-insulin-dependent diabetes is expected to rise as the population ages. You don't have to be among those who spend the rest of their lives monitoring their blood sugar. The keys to the no-diabetes lifestyle are exercise and calorie reduction.

The no-diabetes lifestyle features exercise and a low-calorie diet.

If you're in your forties or early fifties, now is the time to begin the lifestyle changes, like those listed below, that can keep this disease at bay.

Weight control. People usually get diabetes from eating too much and gaining too much weight. Nearly two out of every three diabetics are overweight. If you're obese or have been obese in the past, according to studies conducted at the National Center for Health Services Research, you're roughly two to three times more likely to develop diabetes than others who are slim.

Keep your weight down.

For unknown reasons, people who gain weight in the upper body – who appear barrel chested – are more likely to develop diabetes than people who gain weight in the lower body – who appear bell shaped. But it's clear that weight loss not only reduces the risk of developing diabetes, it also enables many adult-onset diabetics to return to normal blood-sugar metabolism.

Get plenty of exercise.

Exercise. Like weight loss, regular physical exercise can help prevent diabetes. And if you already have the disease, exercise may enable you to manage it without drugs. Inactive older people, according to studies at the National Center for Health Services Research, are three times more likely to develop diabetes than those who get regular exercise.

Staying fit protects against diabetes in several ways. It helps the body metabolize sugar more efficiently by increasing the body's sensitivity to insulin. It also keeps weight down and inhibits the unwanted clumping of blood platelets, which can lead to strokes.

For most healthy people, any kind of aerobic exercise can boost resistance to the disease. For those who have diabetes, exercise should be vigorous, but not jarring. Brisk walking, swimming, and bicycling are ideal. If diabetics take up jogging, they need to check their feet carefully for blisters or cuts, since the disease causes nerve damage that can reduce sensation in the extremities. Of course, any diabetic who wishes to exercise should first consult a physician.

A high-fiber diet may help prevent diabetes.

Dietary fiber. Consuming a diet that's high in fiber may play a role in preventing diabetes. Adding bulk to the digestive tract slows the absorption of sugar through the digestive walls. As a result, sugar levels in the blood stay relatively even and don't overwhelm the body's capacity to handle them.

There are several forms of fiber, however, and not all of them help control diabetes. Oat bran, peas, and other legumes, as well as pectin, a form of fiber found in fruit, all have a stabilizing effect on blood-sugar levels. They contain water-soluble fiber. Other foods that fight diabetes include beans, barley, pasta, parboiled rice, rye bread, pumpernickel bread, and cracked wheat. By contrast, water-insoluble fiber, such as the bran portion of wheat and the cellulose found in most vegetables, promotes regularity, but has little effect on the course of diabetes.

A vegetarian diet. Seventh-Day Adventists, a religious sect, have less than half the mortality rate from diabetes of other white Americans. Their diets may have something to do with it. Adventists typically shun red meat, caffeine, alcohol, and tobacco. Roughly half of them consume a vegetarian diet that allows dairy products and eggs.

After tracking the health histories of almost 26,000 Adventists over a period of 21 years, researchers at the University of Minnesota School of Public Health concluded that their low-meat diets accounted for their low rate of diabetes. Vegetarian diets tend to include more fiber from beans and legumes and contain much less saturated animal fat than the average diet. According to the researchers, saturated fats may adversely affect the function of insulin, and the nitroso compounds found in meats may produce substances known to trigger diabetes in laboratory animals.

Blood pressure control. Though a direct cause and effect relationship has yet to be established, studies suggest that reducing blood pressure may help prevent diabetes. The National Center for Health Services Research study showed that, in the absence of obesity, those whose blood pressures are normal are much less likely to have diabetes than those whose blood pressures are high. This is particularly true for younger people, according to James Anderson, M.D., a fiber and diabetes researcher at the University of Kentucky College of Medicine.

The main elements of diabetes risk reduction are weight control; exercise; a high-fiber, low-saturated-fat diet; and blood-pressure control. These help protect not only against diabetes, but also against its complications: impotence, kidney failure, eye disease, and infections.

Something in the lifestyle of Seventh-Day Adventists offers some protection.

Reducing high blood pressure also may help prevent diabetes.

15

EMOTIONS: THE POWER OF POSITIVE FEELING

The woman rocking back and forth on the porch was petting the neighborhood cat. She rubbed its war-torn ears and stroked the dusty fur until the old warrior's eyes narrowed into slits of gold. A hypnotic purr matched the rhythm of her rocker.

But minutes later the woman changed. The peaceful curves of her face drew down, her fingers tightened on the cat, and the rhythmic rocking stopped. She looked at the cat in astonishment. "What are you doing here?" she exclaimed as she knocked the startled calico to the floor. "Cats give me hives!"

A victim of multiple personality disorder can have one personality that is allergic and one that is not.

The woman, a victim of multiple personality disorder, had changed from one personality to another. And this personality was allergic to cats.

THE FRONTIERS OF MIND/BODY RESEARCH

Even under the extreme mental fractures of a multiple personality, how can one single immune system allow itchy red hives to develop in response to a cat in one personality but no reaction in another? How can the *same* immune system react so differently to a bundle of fur?

This is possible because of connections between the emotions, the brain, and the immune system.

Scientists who are edging along the frontiers of mind/body research at the National Institute of Mental Health are investigating this phenomenon by measuring chemicals that exist within the bloodstream in these patients for only seconds. But the feeling that the answer involves the mechanism by which emotional states directly affect the immune system draws them deeper into a field that has come to be called psychoneuroimmunology – a $12 word that acknowledges the looping connections scientists now see between your emotions, your brain, and your immune system.

No one has mapped out all the underlying pathways that support these connections, but it seems as though your emotions – your responses to the ups and downs of everyday life – are translated by the brain into chemicals. These chemicals have the ability to either suppress or enhance the way your immune system functions. They are apparently messengers that are generated and received by both your brain and your immune system and seem to zip along well-worn pathways between organs and structures that are a part of each system.

The brain translates your emotions into chemicals that communicate with the immune system.

How do these emotion-produced chemicals affect your health? The idea is that negative emotions suppress your immune system, while positive emotions zip it up. So, theoretically at least, if you're hostile or depressed, or afraid, you're more likely to get sick. If you're trusting, caring, or optimistic, you're more likely to stay well.

DEPRESSION CAN BE HAZARDOUS TO YOUR HEALTH

Most of the heavy-duty scientific research across the country has focused on proving the connection between negative emotions and suppression of the immune system, or negative emotions and actual illness or death.

Researchers are examining the connection between negative emotions, illness, and death.

Depressed people seem to experience more illness.

At Mount Sinai School of Medicine in New York, for example, researchers found a link between depression in a group of 15 widowers after their wives' deaths and a significant drop in the ability of their lymphocytes to fight off an invader. In San Diego, U.S. Navy psychologist Ross Vickers, Ph.D., found that depressed recruits were more likely to get a cold during basic training than recruits who demonstrated a more positive emotional state. And in Chicago, a 20-year study of 2,018 electric company workers revealed that depressed employees were almost twice as likely to die of a deadly disease than those with a more positive emotional state.

But some of the most intriguing studies have been conducted by a husband and wife, the immunologist/psychologist team of Janice Kiecolt-Glaser, Ph.D., and Ronald Glaser, Ph.D., at the Ohio State University College of Medicine.

Separation and divorce have an impact on immune function.

The Glasers have pioneered much of the laboratory work that has actually measured the connections between mind, body, and immune system. In one study, for example, they drew blood samples from 38 married women and 38 women who were either separated or divorced. They also gave the women psychological tests that allowed the researchers to define each woman's emotional state. Then, by counting the numbers of microscopic natural killer cells, lymphocytes, and antibodies that rallied to fight off a variety of agents, the Glasers were able to prove two things: that immune function drops immediately after separation or divorce and that women with poor marriages have poor immune function as well. And in both cases, the researchers concluded, the poorer immune function was linked to depression.

HOSTILITY KILLS

Hostility can be hazardous to your health.

Depression is not the only emotion that can be hazardous to your health. Hostility, says

Redford Williams, M.D., director of Duke University's behavioral medical research center, is probably a close second. "It seems pretty clear that you can get significant reductions in immune function when people get hostile," he adds.

How does he know? "We brought people into the lab and harassed them," says Dr. Williams with a chuckle. "And what we found is that people who scored high on a test [of hostility] would get mad. People who scored low [on the test] didn't. Then looking at both kinds of people over a 25-year period, we found that hostile people were five to seven times more likely to die" than people with a more positive way of reacting to the stresses of everyday life.

People who are hostile – people who react to the world as though everyone they meet is personally out to get them – are the ones who get an early flight off the planet.

The same may be true of people who feel they don't "fit in," says J. Stephen Heisel, M.D., a former assistant professor of medicine at Boston University. Dr. Heisel and his colleagues studied 111 healthy college students and found that those who were maladjusted – the ones who felt they didn't "fit in" – had lower numbers of natural killer cells than students who felt comfortable with themselves and their environment.

People who feel they don't "fit in" have lower numbers of natural killer cells.

Moreover, laboratory studies confirm a significant reduction in immune function to a third negative emotion: fear. Donald T. Lysle, Ph.D., a research associate at the University of Pittsburgh Medical School, and his colleagues found that the immune function of laboratory animals – which, in this case, may provide a more accurate measure than studies with people – is reduced by two-thirds when they're afraid.

THE EFFECTS OF BAD EXPERIENCES

But of increasing concern to scientists is not just the fact that negative emotions such as

Immune system changes caused by negative emotions may not be quickly reversed.

depression, hostility, maladjustment, and fear can suppress the immune system. They're also concerned about the possibility that these changes may not be quickly reversed.

When a 6-month-old monkey is separated from its mother, its ability to fight off an infection is reduced tenfold, says Christopher L. Coe, Ph.D., director of the famed primate lab at the University of Wisconsin. Yet even if mother and baby are reunited on the same day, immune function does not return to normal. It stays depressed. And it may stay depressed for weeks or even months, says Dr. Coe.

Bad experiences leave us open to infection and disease for a long time.

What does this phenomenon mean to humans? It may mean that bad experiences leave us open to infection and disease for a long time after the experience, says Dr. Coe.

Everyday worries and disappointments also seem to take their toll.

And it may not take a big-league emotional reaction to trigger a response in your immune system. Everyday worries and disappointments also seem to take their toll. In a study at the State University of New York at Stony Brook, for example, researchers asked 30 students to fill out a four-page psychological questionnaire three times a week and turn it in to the researchers along with a sample of their saliva. The researchers would determine the student's moods from the questionnaire and their antibody levels from the saliva. The result? Antibody levels paralleled their everyday moods, reported the scientists. When the students were down, their antibody levels were down. When they were up, so were their immune defenses.

ACTIVATING THE HEALER WITHIN

Can positive thinking help?

But that study – all the studies in fact – actually raise more questions than they answer. If the immune system is so vulnerable to emotions, can positive emotions counteract the effect of negative ones on your immune system? Can you actually use positive emotions to reprogram your immune system toward maximum effectiveness? Is positive thinking – which is, as the Reverend Norman Vincent Peale has claimed for 30 years, nothing more than making up your mind to exist in a positive emotional state – actually the way to healthful living?

Dr. Peale, author of the bestselling *The Power of Positive Thinking,* says it is. As he notes in his autobiography, *The True Joy of Positive Living:*

> Many years ago I would always develop a horrendous cold in February. It would start with a sore throat, sniffling, aching – all the classic cold symptoms. Inevitably my vocal cords would end up being affected so that I could talk only in a croak. Then I was plunged into a crisis of whether or not I could fill contracted speaking engagements or preach in church on Sunday. Year after year this defeatist situation went on until one day I decided it was irrational and decided to stop it. I realized that there was no sense in the assumption that I must have a cold in February or indeed anytime.
>
> Accordingly, I began to think positively that I need not have such a cold and that I could get through the winter season and never lose my voice, as had been my custom. From the minute I took that firm decision, I have never had another cold, at least, never one that could inhibit activity.

The Reverend Norman Vincent Peale used positive thinking to treat his colds.

Many of us can echo the effectiveness of Dr. Peale's approach to life in general and health in particular. But scientists, who are bound by the laws of physics and their affiliated universities, are more cautious. Some, like Bernie Siegel, M.D., the noted cancer surgeon at Yale University, are willing to say flat out that "positive emotions like love, acceptance, and forgiveness stimulate the immune system." Others, like Steven Locke, M.D., the Harvard University researcher who helped popularize the term *psychoneuroim-*

Scientists are cautious in saying positive thinking might help in healing.

munology, will carefully say, "I believe that under some circumstances, positive expectation and hopefulness and optimism and perhaps even joy and mirth will be shown to be associated with changes in immunity that have some health-promoting powers."

Most scientists want hard data to back them up.

Most scientists seem to agree with Dr. Locke, although they are frequently reluctant to jump up and down on a soap box about it. So even though there's an underground murmur of agreement among the scientific community that a positive emotional state will boost your immune system, most scientists want more hard data before they're willing to promote the idea to the public.

What they are willing to say, however, is that counteracting the negative emotional states induced by depression, maladjustment, fear, and hostility *can* enhance your immune system.

Feeling in control of your life apparently makes a difference.

The key, most seem to agree, is to take charge of your life – to feel that you're in control of your mind, your body, and your environment. "The feeling that you can control what's happening seems to enhance the immune system," confirms David McClelland, Ph.D., a former Harvard University research professor who is now conducting a study on it at Boston University. "We actually have a way to measure that [control], and it clearly predicts less sickness."

COUNTERACTING THE EFFECTS OF FEAR

How do you take charge of your life in a way that will counteract the effects of negative emotions on your immune system? Well, since fear may suppress the immune system, if you have a particular fear that's really bugging you, suggests the University of Pittsburgh's Dr. Lysle, you might check in with a psychologist and work out a program of desensitization.

If you're afraid of bridges, for example, you might start by looking at pictures of bridges, progress to standing under a small one, and end up driving over a big one. The idea, Dr. Lysle explains, is that by increasing your exposure to bridges in a very gradual, controlled manner, the fear will disappear. And you'll have eliminated at least one major immune system suppressant.

If your fear is related to an upcoming event, suggests Robert M. Goisman, M.D., director of the Massachusetts Mental Health Center Phobia Clinic in Boston, you might want to close your eyes and imagine yourself already there. Then play through the situation in your mind: Imagine yourself coping with or even enjoying it. Your imagery will prepare you for the real thing – without fear.

Imagery can help you cope with fears.

S. M. Tweed Culpan, R.N., a clinical nurse specialist who does crisis intervention counseling at the University of Arkansas Medical Center, also uses imagery to help patients reduce fear and gain a sense of control over their lives.

A 51-year-old trucker who was in the medical center to receive skin grafts on his groin, abdomen, and legs, for example, was terrified that the grafts wouldn't take because a previous one had failed. His body's immune system had rejected the graft – treated it as a foreign invader and shot it down. So Culpan, who teaches people to harness their mind and use it as a tool to aid healing, suggested that he develop an image of himself that would maximize his body's efforts at healing.

It seems possible to harness the mind and use it as a tool to aid in healing.

The trucker did. He visualized little guys with feathers who were going to work on the grafts from the inside of his body. They piled the feathers in layers under each graft so that – in the driver's mind – they would make his skin and the graft stick together. And these guys were non-union: they could be called to work

One man used imagery to help skin grafts take.

anytime by a single whistle. A second whistle, the trucker told Culpan, sent the guys back into his body to regenerate.

The grafts took. The trucker's immune system didn't attack the grafts and his body accepted the new skin. How did it work? The physiological messages he was sending to his immune system through imagery were all in the positive vein, Culpan explains. He was programming his emotional state to counteract the negative effects of fear. Moreover, adds Culpan, "We were also using a principle of psychodrama: creativity and anxiety cannot coexist." So while the trucker was creating images, his fear disappeared.

DISARMING HOSTILITY

Eliminating hostility gets rid of a major immune system suppressant.

Another way to take charge of your life and eliminate a major immune system suppressant is to deal with hostility, says Duke University's Dr. Williams, who is author of the forthcoming book *The Trusting Heart.* How do you know if you have any? "The critical thing is if you find yourself getting angry in a lot of trivial situations," says Dr. Williams. "Like getting mad at the people up ahead in traffic jams or lines in a movie theater. When you think about it rationally, they didn't get out of bed with the idea they were going to get you.

"But you can really tell you're hostile if you find yourself imputing evil motives to people," he adds. "If the elevator doesn't come and you find yourself saying, 'Those people up there are just standing there and talking and holding the elevator' when, in reality, you don't know their motives," that's being hostile.

Fortunately, when people recognize their hostility, they can get rid of it. One way is to be more religious, says Dr. Williams. "Every one of the world's religions tells us to treat others the way we want to be treated." If you do that, there's no room in your heart for hostility.

Another way, he adds, is to follow the recommendations made by Meyer Friedman, M.D., the San Francisco cardiologist who first studied behavior marked by impatience, aggressiveness, and hostility, labeled it "Type A," and offered evidence that it may hurt your heart enough to kill you.

"Type-A" behavior may hurt your heart.

Hostility is the part of Type-A behavior that kills, says Dr. Williams. And it doesn't limit its effects to hearts. Through its suppressive effects on your immune system, feelings of hostility are responsible for increasing the death rate *five* to *seven* times among otherwise healthy people.

Fortunately, there are two types of behavioral exercises that can help you exorcise your hostility. The first is general, the second, specific. Perform the general exercises as often as possible on no particular timetable, suggests their creator Dr. Friedman. Do the specific exercises according to schedule – a different exercise once a day for seven days, then repeat the sequence week by week throughout the month. You try a different set of seven exercises for each month. For best results, select specific exercises from the list below and schedule them throughout a full year.

If you're a diehard Type A, these exercises will drive you nuts – at least at first. On the other hand, they can't be any worse than a heart attack or pneumonia.

Perform these exercises to help eliminate Type-A behavior.

GENERAL EXERCISES

Make a concerted effort to do these exercises frequently.

- Announce to your spouse and friends that you intend to turn over a new leaf.
- Start smiling at other people and laughing at yourself.

Smile more, examine your lapses into anger, and learn to listen better.

- Stop trying to think or do more than one thing at a time.
- Play to lose at least some of the time.
- When something angers you, immediately make a note of it. Review the list at the end of each week and decide objectively which items truly merited your level of anger.
- Listen, *really* listen, to the conversation of others.

SPECIFIC EXERCISES

Combine these exercises into seven-day exercises, a different exercise per day, repeating each schedule throughout a month.

- Recall pleasant memories for 15 minutes.
- Don't wear a watch.
- Get in the longest checkout line at the supermarket.
- Do absolutely nothing but listen to music for 15 minutes.
- Buy a small gift for a member of your family.
- Cheerfully say "Good morning" to each member of your family and to people you see at work.

Slow down and smell the roses.

- Carefully, slowly, scrutinize a tree, a flower, the sunset, or dawn.
- Walk, talk, and eat more slowly.
- On two different occasions, say to someone, "Maybe I'm wrong."
- Tape-record your dinnertime conversation, then play back the tape to see whether you interrupt or talk too fast.

BLOCKING HOSTILITY AND DEPRESSION

Use optimism to block hostility and depression.

Another way to eliminate hostility – and depression as well – is to block both emotions with optimism. And, no, that doesn't mean you have to turn yourself into Sally Sunshine. But there's nothing to stop you from using the same coping strategies that optimists naturally apply when something pops up with the potential to send them into a major funk. In fact, it's these strategies, scientists tell us, that apparently block hostility and depression and lead to better health. They may also be the foundation for developing a sense of control over our lives and the key to developing what some scientists have called hardiness.

The foundation of these strategies, reports Michael Scheier, Ph.D., a researcher at Carnegie-Mellon University, is the optimist's natural inclination to meet any problem he runs into head on. Optimists don't waste time denying that a problem exists or worrying about its implications. Instead they identify it, focus on it, deal with it, and make a deliberate attempt to dwell on the good things in any resulting situation.

Optimists accept what they cannot change or control.

This latter strategy also gives the optimist a second advantage, Dr. Scheier suggests. It's the ability to accept what they cannot change or control. Ultimately a pragmatist, the optimist figures there's no sense in getting bent out of shape about something you can't do anything about – a strategy that apparently kicks both hostility and depression right in the teeth.

Scientists are not just guessing about the effects of optimism on health, either. A number of studies, many of them by Dr. Scheier and his University of Miami colleague Charles S. Carver, Ph.D., indicate that optimistic coping strategies are directly related to increased health. A study of 141 college students experiencing end-of-semester turbulence, for example, indicated that optimistic students reported fewer symptoms over a four-week period than students who were not optimistic. And a study of 54 people who underwent heart surgery revealed that optimists healed faster, went home sooner, had fewer complications, and were significantly less likely

Optimists fight off disease better and seem to heal faster.

to experience a heart attack after surgery than pessimists.

How did the patients maintain an optimistic attitude in the face of such a life-threatening event? "Prior to surgery," reported the researchers, "optimists were much more likely to be making plans for themselves and setting goals for their recovery period than were pessimists." And optimists were much less likely to be dwelling on the negative aspects of their emotional experiences – their feelings of nervousness and sadness, for example – than pessimists.

Optimists cope better following surgery.

After surgery, the difference in coping strategies between optimists and pessimists was even more pronounced. Pessimists tried to block out thoughts of what the recovery period might be like, while optimists were trying to gather as much information as possible. Optimists knew they were going home. Pessimists were afraid they weren't.

"To the most basic question – whether there is any evidence that a sense of optimism affected the patient's physical state in any way – the answer is an unqualified yes," the researchers concluded.

USING YOUR SELVES

The more "selves" a person has, the *less* likely negative emotions will affect health.

How else can you take control of your life and boost your immune system? Patricia Linville, Ph.D., an associate professor of psychology at Yale University, has found a link between the number of "selves" you see in yourself and your health. In a study of 106 students, says Dr. Linville, she found that the more roles a student had – wife, mother, student, friend, tennis player, theater buff, lawyer, whatever – the *less* likely negative emotions such as depression were to affect their health. In fact, the "multi-selved" students in her study proved so much less vulnerable to illnesses such as the flu that Dr. Linville suggests we all might be a little more disease resistant if we begin to be more aware of how many selves are actually packaged into a single entity.

The way these selves affect your immune system, Dr. Linville explains, is that both positive and negative emotions are associated with the different selves that make up your personality. So if the self that's a wife is depressed and you see yourself only as a wife, the depression you feel is likely to suppress your immune system and leave you vulnerable to various microorganisms. But if, on the other hand, you also see yourself as a dynamic courtroom lawyer who can take on the world's corporate giants, the positive emotions you feel about that self could actually offset the immune system effects of the depression from your wife role.

The key to counteracting the effect of negative emotions on your immune system, says Dr. Linville, is to concentrate on the selves that are associated with positive emotions. If you're going through a divorce, for example, ignore your wife or husband self and concentrate on your tennis player self – especially if you just beat the pants off the country club pro. If your marriage is just great, thank you, and your tennis game is the pits, think of yourself as "Mary, the great wife," and not "Mary, the lousy tennis player." Then your "great wife" self can block the immune system suppression of the "lousy tennis player" self.

It's not just a case of semantics. It's using your mind to control your emotions. It's the power of positive feeling.

Focus on your best selves in order to counteract the Impact of negative emotions.

16

ENCEPHALITIS:
A FIRE IN THE BRAIN

A female mosquito has just landed on your arm. The female mosquito is a hungry thing. Propelled by the mysterious instinct that drives all life to survive and reproduce, she searches for a meal. In this case, a blood meal, for she must have blood before she lays her eggs.

The type of blood is unimportant. Bird blood is as good as mammal. Yet drinking the blood of other animals can be hazardous. Blood carries nutrients, but it carries other things too. The blood of some birds carries a strange virus.

The encephalitis virus harms neither mosquito nor bird.

Ah, but Mother Nature loves mosquitoes. And she loves birds. This virus harms neither. The mosquito locates a young bird still in the nest and scampers down its unfeathered back. She sinks her slender proboscis beneath the hatchling's skin and drinks its blood, virus and all.

She stores the deadly virus in her gut, where it multiplies. Two weeks later, when its numbers are strong, the virus travels to her salivary glands. Once there, it will remain with her for life, and she will inject it into everything she bites. The female mosquito has become a killer. A female mosquito has just landed on your arm . . .

Encephalitis comes to man either through mosquito bite or herpes simplex 1.

Two major types of encephalitis haunt mankind today, as they have throughout the ages. One is caused by something that happens to almost all of us (mosquito bite), and the other is caused by something almost all of us have (her-

132

pes simplex virus type 1, or HSV-1). Both forms are potentially deadly, have virtually no cure, and are thankfully quite rare – for the most part.

A DIFFERENT KIND OF BITE

Being bitten by a mosquito is something most of us find merely irritating, but a few people will get sick from it. And though most of those will develop a mild form of encephalitis, 1 in 200 will need to be hospitalized. In rare but largely unpredictable instances, some people will suffer severe brain damage and others will die – all from the bite of an infected mosquito. Why some die and others suffer little more than a fever is largely unknown. The immune response seems to be the same in both cases.

Physicians report 1,500 to 2,000 cases of encephalitis annually in the United States, though only 5 to 10 percent are confirmed as such during a typical year. The symptoms of encephalitis are often confused with other diseases, making accurate diagnosis difficult. Sometimes the disease isn't recognized until a mosquito-borne epidemic begins, when hundreds of confirmed cases are reported in different parts of the country.

Diagnosis is difficult; sometimes the disease isn't recognized until an epidemic begins.

The amazing thing is that it doesn't happen more often. Fourteen different strains of virus that cause encephalitis are carried by mosquitoes, of which seven have been observed in North America. Of these, St. Louis encephalitis, California encephalitis, western equine encephalitis, and eastern equine encephalitis are the most active. This unhappy quartet caused nearly 7,000 confirmed cases of encephalitis between 1955 and 1985. If the 200 to 1 ratio of mild to severe cases is applied, possibly 1.4 million Americans contracted some form of mosquito-borne encephalitis during that 30-year period.

Possibly 1.4 million Americans contracted some form of mosquito-borne encephalitis between 1955 and 1985.

DEAD-END HOST

St. Louis and California encephalitis are named after the areas where they were first recognized following major epidemics. The two equine strains earned their names because they were recognized in horses before man. In the days when agriculture depended on horsepower for much of its labor, an outbreak of equine encephalitis was serious business indeed. It was later noticed that the same disease was infecting humans each year at about the same time.

The basic cycle for this virus involves mosquitoes and birds.

Ironically, the virus needs neither horse nor man to survive. "The horse is pretty much a dead-end host, just like humans," says Bruce Francy, Ph.D., chief of the Arbovirus Ecology Branch at the Centers for Disease Control in Ft. Collins, Colorado. "The basic cycle for this virus involves mosquitoes and birds."

The virus, which originates inside birds and small mammals, is spread by mosquitoes.

The virus apparently originates inside the bodies of birds and small mammals and is spread to other birds and small mammals by mosquito *vectors* (disease carriers). Neither the host animals nor the mosquitoes are made ill, and in this manner the virus has been perpetuated throughout time.

When mosquito vectors spread the virus to unprotected people and horses, however, some develop an inflammation of the brain that was called sleeping sickness by earlier generations (it is not related to the African disease, however). We know it today as viral encephalitis.

DESTRUCTIVE RESPONSE

The virus can move across the human blood/brain barrier.

The symptoms of viral encephalitis in humans usually begin three to five days after being bitten. The virus leaves the mosquito's salivary glands, enters its new human host, and travels to the lymph nodes, where it begins replicating. From there it moves to the bloodstream and continues reproducing in different tissues throughout the body. Antibodies in the blood attack the virus, and the battle is joined. If the virus can weather the attack, it will seek out nerve tissue and, through methods still not understood, move across the blood/brain barrier – a network of tightly fused capillaries designed to keep harmful substances from contacting sensitive brain cells.

The blood/brain barrier fails against this foe, however, and once inside the brain the virus invades the delicate neurons and replicates again. This assault signals T-cells, B-cells, and macrophages to respond and attack the infected brain sites. Swelling and inflammation result, but the brain has little room to expand inside the skull and damages itself in the squeeze. Yet the immune system battles on, determined to wipe out the invader at any cost. B-cells launch antibodies to mark the spreading virus, T-cells puncture and destroy infected brain matter, and macrophages mop up the aftermath.

The brain swells, expands against the skull, and is damaged.

A similar battle waged against antigens invading a skinned knee would result in minor inflammation, a scab, and perhaps a small scar. But this is not a knee, and while seeking to rid the brain of its infection, the immune system can propel an encephalitis victim toward permanent brain damage or death.

The damage being done inside the skull doesn't take long to surface. "The primary symptoms are severe, excruciating headache and stiff neck," says Paul McKinney, M.D., an internist at the Medical College of Wisconsin. Changes in mental status soon follow, he says, including confusion, disorientation, and hallucinations. "It appears sometimes like a stroke, and seizures may develop. It's the type of thing where a person would be hospitalized fairly soon."

Symptoms are severe.

Hospital care, however, is what's known to physicians as "supportive," that is, it's designed to keep the patient alive while the virus runs its

Hospital care is supportive; antiviral drugs can't help.

course. "The treatment consists of giving drugs to reduce the swelling in the brain," says Dr. Francy. Physicians also administer drugs to reduce the fever, because victims in fatal cases typically develop fevers of 106° F or more. "Other than that there's nothing else to do. There are no antiviral drugs for this disease."

RISKY BUSINESS

Vaccines exist but are not available to the American public.

Antiviral drugs to help the body fight off an attack of encephalitis may not be available, but vaccines capable of protecting humans from this disease do exist – they just aren't made available to the public.

Dr. McKinney suggested in a *New England Journal of Medicine* article in 1988 that visitors to the Olympic Games in Seoul, Korea, be vaccinated against Japanese encephalitis, a potent strain that produces 10,000 cases in Asia every year and boasts a grim fatality rate of 50 percent or more. The U.S. government, however, would not agree to protect the vaccine manufacturer against lawsuits that might arise from an inoculation program (remember swine flu?). So American athletes and their families traveled to Korea at their own risk.

Japanese school children have access to vaccines; so do American horses.

The Japanese encephalitis vaccine is routinely administered to Japanese schoolchildren, however, and has been credited with significantly reducing outbreaks in that country. And the U.S. Department of Defense protects the vaccine manufacturer against litigation so that American servicemen and government workers can receive protection before assignment to Asian posts. American tourists, though, are merely advised to carry insect repellent.

Closer to home, "experimental" vaccines are used to protect laboratory workers from western and eastern equine encephalitis, and commercially available vaccines protect horses. No such protection is afforded the general public, however, and it seems unlikely that any vaccine will be offered in the near future. "It's not something a commercial pharmaceutical company would be interested in," says Dr. Francy. "There isn't a market for it, and nobody, including the government, is interested in a vaccine that would be of such limited use – especially with the liability problems involved in that sort of thing."

WHAT CAN BE DONE?

Yet the public is not left completely unprotected. The term *viral encephalitis,* combined with the chilling word "epidemic," sends shivers of fear through the hearts of public health officials coast to coast.

Small wonder. Tracing the history of St. Louis encephalitis back to the mid-1970s, we find a dozen outbreaks and 2,268 cases between 1974 and 1976. Since then, outbreaks have followed in Florida (1977), Mississippi (1979), New Orleans (1980), Texas (1980 and 1986), Southern California (1983 through 1986), and Colorado (1985). And that's just one strain.

Outbreaks of viral encephalitis are not uncommon.

So it comes as no surprise that health officials diligently keep tabs on this disease. What may prove surprising is the rather strange methods they employ to monitor the status of the disease inside our nation's mosquitoes. Robert Wallis, Ph.D., a professor of medical entomology at the Yale University School of Medicine, explains one method – the "sentinel flock."

"Some poultry farmers raise pheasants, and after the young hatch they are kept in open pens during late spring." he says. "Since the ringed-neck pheasant is native to China and has no immunities to our encephalitis strains, there's a high incidence of mortality if the mosquitoes

Ringed-neck pheasants provide an early warning.

that bite them are infected." That information is passed on to public health officials, who begin scouring the area for more evidence of infection. Chickens are also used as sentinels, and the percentage of birds infected in an area gives a clue to the transmission rate and magnitude of a possible outbreak.

Does that mean the health and safety of countless American citizens depends on flocks of pheasants and chickens?

There is only one known preventive for viral encephalitis: avoiding mosquito bites.

"Right," says Dr. Wallis. "They give health officials some warning ahead of time so the population can be advised to take precautions by utilizing repellent, wearing protective clothing, and avoiding outside activity right after dusk, which is when mosquitoes do most of their biting." Apparently, avoiding mosquito bites is the only known method for preventing viral encephalitis.

A couch potato lifestyle protects against the disease.

And, ironically, research has shown that a laid-back, couch potato lifestyle may do more to protect Americans from encephalitis than all the pheasants in China. Scientists recently surveyed places in California, for example, where outbreaks of encephalitis had once been annual events, but they found virtually no cases at all today.

"The reason is a change in lifestyle," Dr. Wallis explains. "In the early 1950s, only one family out of 50 had a TV set, and none of them had air conditioning in their homes. When they came home from work they sat out on the porch and talked, or maybe they had a cookout that lasted into the evening. The mosquitoes ate 'em up, and we had encephalitis every year."

Now, he says, surveys show that all the homes in these areas have TVs, and most have air conditioning, too. "Today they come home from work, stay inside, and watch TV," says Dr. Wallis. "They don't get bitten – and they don't get encephalitis."

WHEN HERPES CAN KILL

If you've ever had a fever blister, you're at risk for herpes simplex encephalitis (HSE), a disease that, for all intents and purposes, erupts as a blister in your brain instead of on your lip.

It is frightening not in the number of victims claimed, for these are relatively few, but in the number of potential victims from which it has to choose, which are millions.

For those of us who've had a fever blister and thus know ourselves to be infected with herpes simplex virus type 1, our only consolation lies in the odds. No more than 1,000 to 2,000 cases of HSE are diagnosed annually. But long-shot odds against becoming a victim must remain our only source of consolation, for there is nothing that places one HSV-1 carrier at greater or lesser risk than any other. HSE is an equal-opportunity infection.

REALM OF UNCERTAINTY

For those who rub their unblemished upper lip and breathe easier for it, be advised that 90 percent of all adults have been exposed to HSV-1 and likely harbor the virus. Only the 25 percent of us who've suffered a fever blister know for sure where we stand.

And we stand in the great realm of medical uncertainty. More is unknown than known about HSE – though what has been learned is as fascinating as it is frightening.

Richard Dix, M.D., a virologist at the University of Miami School of Medicine, is clearly fascinated. Like many researchers across the land, Dr. Dix and his colleagues continue searching for keys to unlock the mystery of HSE, though it's clear they have a long way to go. At present, they really aren't sure how the disease comes about, and they have no idea why you might get a fever blister this month, only to come down

If you've ever had a fever blister, you are at risk for another kind of encephalitis.

Scientists have not unlocked the connections between herpes simplex and encephalitis.

with encephalitis next month. All they know is that the two may be related somehow.

"When you're exposed to HSV-1 as a child," Dr. Dix explains, "it will remain latent in the nerve that supplies sensation to your mouth. When the virus reactivates, it will usually travel down that nerve and produce a fever blister."

Some researchers believe the virus makes a wrong turn on its way to the lip and enters the brain instead.

But when it comes to HSE, some researchers believe the virus makes a wrong turn on its way to the lip and enters the brain instead. "I don't believe that," says Dr. Dix, "because there's something like 98 million cases of fever blister a year in this country, and only about 1,000 to 2,000 cases of encephalitis."

Dr. Dix believes that with 98 million HSV-1 viruses traveling the nerve pathway to the lip every year, more wrong turns would be made – if wrong turns explained encephalitis.

Then again, the virus may gain entry to the brain through the nose.

"I think what really happens," he says, "and we're exploring this in the lab right now, is that the virus gains entry to the brain through the nose. From there it travels up to the olfactory bulb [the nerves located on the underside of the brain that give us our sense of smell] and into the brain and causes encephalitis."

That theory is a radical departure from the accepted view that HSE is caused by an HSV-1 virus gone bad. But there's little comfort to be gained from this new school of thought. If correct, HSE would then become a primary disease instead of a reactivated one, "and you would catch it by being in the wrong place at the wrong time," Dr. Dix says. "I'm not sure how it would occur . . . perhaps if somebody sneezed in your face."

MORE CERTAINTY, MORE FEAR

Mosquito-borne encephalitis and the disease caused by herpes are quite dissimilar.

Except for the inflammation that takes place in the brain, HSE bears little resemblance to its mosquito-borne cousin, viral encephalitis. (Though both are caused by a virus, only the latter is so named.) Unlike viral encephalitis, the

HSE virus does not move through the bloodstream, traveling instead along pathways of nerves. Since it is not transmitted by mosquitoes, there have been no outbreaks or epidemics, and this is good. HSE can be even harder to diagnose than viral encephalitis. Because it travels nerve pathways instead of through the blood, brain biopsy remains the only certain way to diagnose HSE.

Despite those differences, the destruction that takes place in the brain is quite similar in both diseases, as are their outward symptoms. "The early onset of the disease is marked by a headache, and then maybe some personality changes," says Dr. Dix. "The patient will then go into some paralysis or seizures, possibly, and that's when they're usually brought to the emergency room. They may become comatose soon after that."

The brain destruction they cause *is* similar.

Without proper treatment, the period of time between onset and death is about ten days. "It's a fast disease," says Dr. Dix.

Fortunately, acyclovir – the same drug used to control outbreaks of genital herpes (HSV-2) – has proven an effective antiviral treatment for HSE. Injections are given instead of pills, however, and treatment must begin immediately. Patients who are already comatose when first treated often suffer permanent brain damage and fare poorly, regardless of treatment used.

Quick treatment with acyclovir can help victims of HSE.

Since quick diagnosis is the key, one wonders how many physicians would be able to recognize this rare disease on sight? "A lot of things mimic herpes encephalitis, but if you're at a medical center with a good neurologist on board, he will pick it up," says Dr. Dix.

Rapid diagnosis is vital, but doctors may not recognize the disease.

And acyclovir is "a clever drug," he notes. "What you want to do is knock out the virus without killing the cell. Acyclovir does this by targeting the specific proteins of the virus, not those of the brain cell, making it less destructive than earlier antiviral drugs used to combat the disease.

"Treatment can now be a bit more aggressive," he adds. "Even if we're uncertain of the diagnosis, acyclovir is not very toxic, so we tend to put the patient on it and see what happens."

WHO SURVIVES?

You have a better chance of survival if you're under 30.

Age and luck largely determine who survives an HSE attack. "The cutoff point is about 30 years of age," says Dr. Dix. After that, your chances of recovery dwindle. Recovery also depends on how soon the acyclovir is administered. "You want to get it early, while you're still in the headache or seizure stage," he says. "A great deal depends on the knowledge of the physician who sees you when you're admitted to the hospital."

Even so, Dr. Dix notes that many patients suffer irreversible brain damage and must be institutionalized.

With such a poor prognosis, are chances for prevention any better? "There's probably no way you can protect yourself from this disease by boosting your immune system," says Dr. Dix.

Boosting your immune system to fight this disease would be disastrous.

In fact, he says, that's half the problem. "If a virus that's not supposed to be there enters the brain, a strong, healthy immune system is going to come in and say, 'Let's clear this virus out.' Well, in doing so, it starts killing off cells and causes destruction of the brain."

Remarkably, tragically perhaps, patients suffering from AIDS are probably safest of all from this disease, as Dr. Dix discovered early in his career. "I did my training in San Francisco," he says, "and we started seeing the first AIDS patients while I was there. We noticed that those who had HSE showed a different, milder pattern of disease." That's small consolation from an immune-system trade-off few if any of us would ever choose to make.

17

EPSTEIN-BARR VIRUS: AN EPIDEMIC OF FATIGUE

"God gives me strength as I need it," says Janet Bohanon, a 48-year-old Kansas City mother who is forced to spend 22 hours a day in bed. And she isn't talking muscle power.

Epstein-Barr virus made one woman pray for strength.

She means a down-and-dirty, shovel-it-out emotional strength that allows her to sit – or more often lie – calmly at the epicenter of a medical storm. It's a storm that whips her with cruel labels – liar, fake, bum – and rocks her with controversy. Because Janet Bohanon – former model, grocery-store owner, swimmer, tennis player, and all-around mom – is infected with the Epstein-Barr virus (EBV).

How does she know? She's had a diagnosis. She's had blood tests. She has a support group of 10,000 people across the country who all say they have the same thing. But some people – doctors included – say she doesn't. They say she's lazy. Or crazy. Or part of a family of hypochondriacs.

She joined a support group to see her through.

"Yes," she chuckles tiredly, "one doctor actually said that to my face. I spent 3 years in bed when it first hit, my daughter – my daughter who got straight A's and never missed a day of school – had to drop out of school because she got EBV, too. I lost a big house in the suburbs. I lost $60,000 a year in income. And all because I'm 'lazy.' It's been like a nightmare," she sighs. "A nightmare that's lasted for 13 years."

A VIRUS THAT LIVES FOREVER

Most of us carry Epstein-Barr virus but don't get seriously infected.

What is Epstein-Barr? It's a virus that most of us carry in the epithelial lining of the nose and throat. Most children have it by the age of 10 or 11, says Neil Cooper, M.D., a member of the Research Institute of Scripps Clinic in California, although in industrialized countries where we're able to limit our contact with dirt and germs, some of us escape. We don't get seriously infected with the virus, however, unless it hits us as an acute attack of infectious mononucleosis – yep, the kissing disease – in high school or maybe college.

The virus invades the immune system and makes the immune cells fight each other.

The virus invades the B-cells of the immune system itself and sets up what one scientist describes as a state of "civil war." It's a civil war because it essentially pits one set of immune system warriors against another. The immune system's natural killer cells, cytotoxic and suppressor T-cells, plus a variety of antibodies, hunt down the same immune system's virus-infected B-cells.

It's brother against brother at the cellular level. But the war is never won – or lost. Even when the EBV-infected B-cells are gone, they're far from vanquished. A few B-cells always manage to escape the surveillance of your immune system's T-cell defense and hide.

Where? "There's some evidence that the viruses sit in the epithelial cells in the nasopharynx," says David A. Thorley-Lawson, Ph.D., an EBV researcher at Tufts University. They don't cause any symptoms, but when the epithelial cells move to the surface of the epithelium that lines your nose and throat – a natural part of cellular development – they mature. And maturity apparently triggers the virus to replicate – as though you were being constantly reinfected.

"The epithelium," says Dr. Thorley-Lawson "is a well from which the virus can be drawn forever."

The only time the "well" seems to pose a life-threatening danger is if you live in Africa or southern China. In these countries, the infection is associated with a form of nose and throat cancer that, in China at least, is the first or second most frequent cause of death.

In China and Africa, the infection can be fatal.

No one knows why the cancer is as common there as it is rare here, but scientists at Ohio State University have recently discovered that the transformation of EBV into a cancer-causing agent seems to take place only in the presence of certain chemicals found in traditional Chinese herbal medicines that contain the plants from the families *Euphorbiaceae* and *Thymelaeaceae* – known in the United States as varieties of spurge, daphne, mezereon, hogwort, croton, poinsettia, crown-of-thorns, snow-on-the-mountain, tung-oil tree, pencil tree, and candelabra. The plants, unfortunately, are common in southern China.

Certain traditional Chinese herbs turn the virus into a cancer-causing menace.

FEVERS, SORE THROATS, AND MALAISE

Childhood symptoms of an EBV infection are so mild that they usually go unnoticed. They include a slight sore throat, a little tiredness, maybe a day of fever. "You might think you had a cold or the flu," says Scripps' Dr. Cooper.

A childhood infection is mild, but in adults the infection takes the form of mono.

The symptoms of mono, however, are hard to miss: high fever, sore throat, swollen glands, headache, weakness, and a fatigue so devastating you can hardly lift your head. Most cases don't require treatment, and aspirin, bed rest, and salt-water gargles will commonly relieve the symptoms. Mono usually lasts from one to four weeks, although it has been known to persist for several months.

Some people simply can't shake the infection.

And therein lies the controversy that surrounds Janet Bohanon and others like her. Some people never seem to get rid of it. Or it lasts years instead of months. Or it waxes and wanes, gone one day and back the next – reactivated by some unknown factor.

When this happens, some doctors diagnose it as active Epstein-Barr or chronic Epstein-Barr. Others call it chronic mononucleosis. Still others call it a crock.

The controversy centers around the fact that anyone who has ever been infected by the Epstein-Barr virus always will show evidence of infection, and the tests designed to detect somewhat elevated levels of these antibodies are, as one researcher puts it, "meaningless."

Researchers doubt that Epstein-Barr is responsible for all the symptoms laid at its door.

EBV antibody levels can be elevated by *many* things, not just by EBV. "A lot of nonspecific stress can raise your EBV antibodies," explains Ben Katz, M.D., an assistant professor of infectious diseases at Yale University. "And if you get sick, your antibody count goes up. But the increased antibody activity won't cause symptoms and doesn't indicate an active EBV infection."

That's not to say the symptoms of this condition don't exist. They do. Particularly the fatigue. "I believe the symptoms of fatigue are clearly real," says Robert Schooley, M.D., an assistant professor of medicine at Harvard University. "These are not lazy people. These are, if anything, overachievers who suddenly hit a wall and can't function."

EBV *can* be reactivated by a severely suppressed immune system.

In a few rare cases, the cause of fatigue has been determined. EBV *can* be reactivated by a severely suppressed immune system, says Yale's Dr. Katz. "I'm talking about big-league immuno-suppression," he says. "Not the kind from [a poor] diet. Not from stress. If you have AIDS, if you're having an organ transplant and doctors are giving you immunosuppressive drugs, that's the kind of immunosuppression I'm talking about."

Giovanna Tosato, M.D., an EBV investigator for the Food and Drug Administration, agrees. "Minor, transient immunosuppression wouldn't reactivate the virus," she says. "The condition occurs only because of congenital or drug-induced severe immunodeficiencies, or a genetic defect of the T-cells. You really have to be totally deficient. This is one of the last immune functions of the T-cells to go."

Minor, transient immunosuppression won't reactivate the virus.

CHRONIC FATIGUE SYNDROME

So what is it when an attack of mono seems to go on and on? The answer may lie with a newly discovered virus called human B-cell lymphotropic herpes virus (HBLV). "When the dust settles," says Dr. Schooley, "it's possible that what we'll find is that in some of these people HBLV – or maybe some other agent – is playing a role. You could even work up a scenario where HBLV decreases immune response and reactivates EBV."

When an attack of mono just won't quit, the real culprit may be a newly discovered virus.

This possibility explains why researchers across the country have renamed chronic EBV chronic fatigue syndrome (CFS). It's a working title for research purposes, scientists say, and it opens the way for an open-minded look at what causes the chronic fatigue problem.

But while a new name validates the fatigue, fever, sore throats, and headaches of people who suffer from CFS, it's still just a name.

"People want somebody to do something other than saying, 'You're tired and I don't know why,'" says Dr. Schooley. "Unfortunately, right now, I think that's the most honest and the fairest thing to do.

Beware of bizarre treatments offered for EBV.

"Stay out of the hands of people who do dramatic things," he cautions those who have the syndrome. "There are a lot of people who are doing a lot of bizarre things that range all the way from colonic irrigation to immunoglobulin therapy. Instead, maximize your productivity [during the times] you're feeling well."

Janet Bohanon agrees. "I've *got* to be worthwhile," she says. So during the 2 hours a day she's not in bed, she directs regional efforts of the National Chronic Fatigue Syndrome Association – formerly the National Chronic Epstein-Barr Virus Association. She answers telephone queries from across the country and as far away as Australia. She plans community education projects. She writes letters. She keeps up with the medical literature that discusses chronic fatigue and Epstein-Barr.

One long-term sufferer advises prioritizing your life.

You've got to prioritize your life, Bohanon says. When you have barely enough energy to breathe, you learn to decide what's important and let the rest of the world go hang.

If you don't like doing housework – and she doesn't – you don't do it. "Give yourself permission to leave your chores," she says. "Don't push. Learn to ask for help and let your family and friends do the grocery shopping, the cooking, and the cleaning."

Keep your mind busy when your body is inactive.

And when you're confined to bed, keep your mind busy. Watch old movies on a VCR. Take up a low-energy hobby like crocheting. Listen to call-in shows on the radio where people argue passionately over public issues.

Above all, she adds, learn to accept your illness. Learn to accept the fact that a person's worth is not based on a blood test. Learn to accept *yourself.*

18

EXERCISE:
IT'S GOOD FOR WHAT AILS YOU

One, two, three, four . . . Bet you thought you were just exercising your muscles, huh?

You didn't realize your lymphocytes were out there running around that track with you? Or that your neutrophils were bicycling along that woodland path? Or that your macrophages joined in when you swam those laps?

Researchers have been putting the various components of the immune system through their paces, trying to figure out just what happens to your infection-fighting machinery when you work out. They peer at blood, sweat, and saliva through microscopes. They study the disease profiles of active, athletic populations versus inactive, couch potato populations. They expose exercising lab animals to infections. Researchers test and they measure and they prod and they poke. And they've found out that a whole lot happens to your immune system when you exercise.

Ah, but what does it all mean? Do push-ups empower your T-cells? Do your killer cells kill better if you do aerobic dance? Can jogging sharpen your antibodies' microbe-zapping abilities? There's the rub. The researchers don't know. They just don't know whether all the fascinating things they see happening on the cellular level mean anything at all. But they keep looking. They keep on experimenting.

Components of your immune system come along for the ride when you exercise.

Your immune system undergoes a lot of changes when you exercise.

Researchers don't know what all the changes mean.

SO WHY SWEAT?

"Exercise is something that *should* rev up your immune system," says Matthew Kluger, Ph.D., professor of physiology at the University of Michigan Medical School.

It seems logical that exercise might benefit your immune system.

Looking at everything else that regular exercise does for the human body, it would seem logical that it might help keep the immune system in shape as well, but the experimental data just don't support that. Yet.

Moderate exercise may help your infection-fighting abilities.

Some animal experiments seem to indicate that moderate exercise may help your infection-fighting abilities, says Dr. Kluger. He describes one study in which animals allowed access to an exercise wheel fared better when exposed to infection than their sedentary counterparts.

His own experiments with humans have shown that exercise increases the levels of certain infection-fighting white cells in the blood. The amount of endogenous pyrogen, the chemical you produce during fevers, also goes up. Your body temperature increases somewhat immediately following a workout, but that is probably due to heat produced by working muscles rather than the presence of these chemicals, says Dr. Kluger.

Other studies, small and inconclusive for the most part, have found a number of other postexercise effects on the immune system. The numbers of various types of white blood cells go up and in some cases their functioning is enhanced. Be aware, however, that some studies have suggested that the numbers of these key infection-fighting cells take a nosedive following excessive exercise.

Population studies show that people who exercise regularly may be less likely to get cancer.

Some population studies, however, give you a really good immunological reason to exercise. People who exercise regularly may be less likely to get cancer. One study that questioned more than 5,000 women college graduates found that students who participated in college sports had a lower lifetime cancer rate than nonathletes. Nonathletes faced almost twice the risk of breast cancer and more than double the amount of cancer of the reproductive system as did the athletes.

Although the findings are not unusual, the people conducting the cancer studies can't figure out what it is about exercise that seems to be doing the trick. Perhaps it's because exercise helps keep obesity at bay, and there is a strong link between obesity and some forms of cancer.

Is it the exercise itself or the exercisers' healthy lifestyle that offers protection?

On the other hand, people who exercise regularly also tend to make other changes in their lives that might play a role in lessening their risk of cancer. They make changes in their diets. They stop smoking. Researchers can't tell whether the reduced cancer risk comes from the direct effects that exercise has on the immune system or from such positive lifestyle changes.

EXERCISE ANYWAY

Okay, so no one has yet determined how exercise makes one bit of difference to your immune system. The evidence is still undeniable that regular exercise is good for your health, says Harvey Simon, M.D., assistant professor of medicine at Harvard Medical School and a member of the Cardiovascular Health Center and Infectious Disease Unit at Massachusetts General Hospital in Boston.

Exercise is good for your health in any case.

But how regular? Should you exercise when you're feeling crummy? When you're sick?

If you're feeling under the weather and the problem is an upper respiratory infection with sniffles and other mild cold symptoms, it's okay to exercise, advises Dr. Simon.

You should avoid exercise when you have a fever.

The one time you *really* want to avoid exercise is when you have a fever. Animal studies suggest that exercising when you have a fever may lead to myocarditis, an inflammation of the heart that is sometimes fatal. Myocarditis is a recognized cause of death in young military recruits, who must frequently exercise whether they feel up to it or not. The dangers of exercising during fever are not to be taken lightly, says Dr. Simon.

And many athletes avoid exercise when they aren't well because their coordination and form are off and they just don't get a training effect.

Exercising regularly will certainly boost your health. The intricacies of how working out may or may not rev up your immune system have yet to be explained. Nevertheless, here's the bottom line: Exercise helps keep you healthy.

19

FEVER: HEALING HEAT

You have a thermostat in your head. In many ways it's like the one that works the furnace in your home.

Set at a nice toasty 98.6° F, give or take a degree or two depending upon the time of day, your internal thermostat works to keep your body temperature constant. Whether you're trudging through slush or baking yourself brown on a tropical beach, your thermostat is quietly making its hormonal adjustments. You shiver. You sweat. You pull off a sweater or throw a shawl over your shoulders. No matter. Your temperature stays the same.

Your internal thermostat maintains your temperature at a constant level.

"No one knows exactly how it works, but it behaves in every way like a thermostat," says Elisha Atkins, M.D., retired Yale University professor of medicine who made research on fever his life's work. "It's in the base of the brain, in the animal part of the brain called the hypothalamus. That's down below where people do their thinking."

When you want to turn up the heat in your house you reach over, give the dial a twist, and the furnace kicks on. Inside your body, it's your immune system that presses the right buttons to fan the flames of fever.

Your immune system can reset the thermostat.

STARTING THE SIZZLE

During an infection, micro-organisms release toxins known as pyrogens.

During an infection, which is the most common cause of fever, invading microorganisms release certain toxins into your body. These toxins are known as pyrogens. The word "pyrogen," explains Dr. Atkins, comes from the Greek words for "create" and "fire." And that's just what these toxins do when they come in contact with your monocytes, the "garbage-eating" immune cells that are just hanging around in your body waiting for action.

Cells of your immune system apparently turn up your thermostat in response to these toxins.

When the monocytes encounter invading organisms or their toxic products, the whistle blows in their little chemical factories – and they fight fire with fire. One of the proteins they start to make is endogenous pyrogen, your very own internal fire-making substance, which is also known as interleukin-1 (IL-1). Scientists believe that the IL-1 sloshing around in your bloodstream turns up the thermostat in your hypothalamus, which then makes you shiver until the tiny muscular movements raise your temperature to the designated level. Then, IL-1 also stimulates your lymphocytes to produce antibodies against infection.

"The really amazing thing about all this is that your lymphocytes produce antibodies much more effectively at the temperature at which interleukin-1 sets the body," says Dr. Atkins.

So your immune system manufactures a chemical substance that both stimulates antibody production and sets the temperature that enhances that antibody production. That's one talented chemical. In addition, the elevated temperature dilates blood vessels, which helps antibodies move into the spaces between the body organ's cells.

It's better to let a low-grade fever run its course.

When you interfere with fever by taking medications to reduce your temperature, you may actually be blocking one of the infection-fighting mechanisms of your immune system, says Dr. Atkins. In general, the best thing to do for low-grade fever is to let it run its course.

"Fever is controlled. Remember, you have a thermostat, and it's not dangerous to set your thermostat up, because your thermostat never goes above 106°F," says Dr. Atkins. "Like everything else in medicine, there are trade-offs. You don't want somebody with a poor heart or poor lungs to raise the body temperature up to 103° or 104°F because that makes the heart work faster and the blood pressure is likely to go up a bit."

Fever in children, who are liable to have fever-caused seizures at higher temperatures, is another matter. When a child's fever reaches 104°F, it's definitely time for concern.

Fever in children, the elderly, and people with heart conditions may be cause for concern.

Dr. Atkins advises fever reduction for the elderly, people with high blood pressure or heart disease, and young children. But any fever may be serious, so it's most important to consult a doctor for diagnosis and treatment – such as getting a prescription for antibiotics to treat a bacterial infection.

The best means for reducing fever is still aspirin or acetaminophen (such as Tylenol) for adults and acetaminophen for children. (Children who have fever should never be given aspirin because it has been linked to Reye's Syndrome.)

Temperatures above 106°F mean that something besides fever is going on, says Dr. Atkins. Heatstroke can cause such high temperatures, as can a disorder of the hypothalamus caused by a stroke or a blow to the head. Fever-reducing medications will not work in such cases. Elevated temperatures caused by these factors are medical emergencies and must be treated in the hospital.

When mildly elevated temperatures are caused by a viral infection, the best thing you can do (after consulting a doctor) is give your immune system a boost by letting well enough alone, advises Dr. Atkins.

20

FOOD POISONING: FIVE EASY WAYS TO AVOID IT

You cut up a raw chicken on a wooden cutting board. Then you cut up vegetables for a salad, using the same knife and cutting board. Can you spot the three mistakes that could send you to the bathroom with diarrhea – or even to the hospital?

Improper treatment of raw chicken can make you sick.

Raw chicken frequently harbors bacteria. When you cut it up, bacteria get on your hand and on your knife and soak into the porous cutting board. If you then use your hands, your knife, and the cutting board to prepare a salad, the bacteria are transmitted to the vegetables you're tossing in the bowl. And that's going to make you sick.

Reactions to the bacteria that grow on chicken range from diarrhea to death.

When the kind of bacteria that grows on chicken hits your digestive tract, the toxic waste products it creates frequently cause diarrhea, cramps, and vomiting. Occasionally, they can kill. Fortunately, your immune system usually keeps the effects of a bacterial invasion confined to a brief bout of illness. Your B-cells order out your antibody warriors to track down the bacterial toxins that are making you sick, lock on to the intruders, and call in a part of the immune system called complement to punch holes in the evildoers – a process that effectively kills them. Then your antibodies go after the bacteria themselves and prevent them from multiplying. It may take a while, sometimes even weeks, but eventually all the bacteria are destroyed.

There are more than 1,800 strains of salmonella bacteria, and most of them can cause
food poisoning. But there are other culprits,
too. *Staphylococcus aureus, Clostridium botu-
linum,* and *Clostridium perfringens* are three of
the most well known. And all can make you sick
anytime from 1 hour to several days after you've
eaten them. Staphylococcus may cramp you into
a fetal position between 1 and 6 hours after a
meal, while salmonella may take a few days.

Salmonella is not the only cause of food poisoning.

Unfortunately, all four of these bacteria are
everywhere. Most fish and poultry, for example,
are contaminated by salmonella before they even
get to your home. So rather than trying to get rid
of these bacteria – actually an impossible task –
preventing their growth or killing them before
they attack is the only way you can protect
yourself. Here are five easy ways to do it.

The culprits are everywhere, and you need to take steps to protect yourself.

KEEP IT COLD OR KEEP IT HOT

Improper holding temperature is responsible for most reported cases of food poisoning.
"Many illnesses come from church picnics, where
the food is prepared earlier, taken out, and held
for hours," says Tom Schwarz, assistant director for program development in the retail-food
protection branch of the Food and Drug Administration.

Most bacteria are killed by temperatures
above 165°F. They are prevented from growing
at temperatures above 150°F or below 40°F.
But in between, they grow very quickly (the
warmer, the quicker). Keep food at those in-
between temperatures and you're looking for
trouble, especially if you hold it for more than
2 hours.

It's unwise, for example, to let a hot dish
cool on the counter before putting it in the

refrigerator. As it gradually cools, it spends a lot of time in the optimum temperature range for bacteria growth. "The aim is to cool food to 40° within 4 hours," says Schwarz. The food will cool off much more quickly in the refrigerator.

Watch that stuffing—don't give salmonella a warm place to nest.

But you have to use common sense, too. Even refrigeration won't save you from the toxic effects of a turkey stuffed the night before Christmas. While it may seem as though nothing is stirring, not even a mouse, the salmonella in your bird are probably throwing a party. They're throwing a party because raw turkeys harbor salmonella. And if you pack a bird tightly with warm stuffing, the bacteria will have all night to multiply. Even though it's refrigerated, the cold just can't penetrate to the center of the turkey fast enough. So refrigerate only an *un*stuffed bird, and cook the stuffing separately.

Thaw frozen meat in the refrigerator.

Take care to keep raw foods refrigerated as well. If a piece of meat is contaminated with staphylococcus (there's no way to know if it is) and it sits at room temperature for hours, the meat may be loaded with toxin by the time you cook it. And the toxin is not destroyed by heating.

That's why you should think far enough ahead to thaw foods in the refrigerator. If you must leave them out, thaw them in sealed packaging under cold water. And try to have the refrigerator door open as briefly and infrequently as possible, to make sure it stays at 40° F.

Molds can invade the refrigerator.

The one instance where keeping foods cold isn't also going to keep them safe is with mold. Molds grow in the refrigerator because they can tolerate the low temperature. And under the right conditions, they can produce mycotoxins, or poisons.

What should you do if the fuzzies pay a visit to your refrigerator? Here are some recommendations from the U.S. Department of Agriculture.

Don't sniff the moldy item – molds can cause respiratory problems. If the food is heavily covered with mold, wrap it gently and discard it immediately. Clean the refrigerator where the food was sitting and examine nearby items.

If the food has only a tiny spot of mold, proceed as follows:

- In hard block cheeses, cut off at least an inch around and below the mold spot. Keep your knife out of the mold. Rewrap in fresh wrap. The same procedure can be followed for hard salami and smoked turkey.
- In jams and jellies, a tiny spot of mold can be scooped out. With a second, clean spoon, scoop out more jam around the spot. If the rest looks and smells normal, it's okay. If it tastes fermented, throw it out.
- In firm vegetables, such as cabbage and carrots, you can cut away small spots of mold from the surface. But you should discard soft vegetables – tomatoes, cucumbers, and lettuce, for example – if they show mold growth.
- Discard moldy soft cheese, cottage cheese, cream, sour cream, yogurt, individual cheese slices, bacon, hot dogs, sliced lunch meats, meat pies, opened canned ham, baked chicken, bread, cake, buns, pastry, corn, nuts, flour, whole grains, rice, dried peas and beans, and peanut butter.

Lop mold off cheeses and scoop it out of jams.

Some moldy foods can be saved, but others must be tossed.

COOK IT WELL

You can avoid a lot of problems by thoroughly cooking meat, poultry, and seafood, which are frequently contaminated with various bacteria. As a general rule, cooking those foods to an internal temperature of 165°F should kill any freeloading bacteria. That goes for leftovers as

Cook meat enough to kill bacteria and parasites.

well. And they should be reheated to 165°F, not just warmed up.

Tasting foods while they're cooking is also hazardous. So-called Jewish mothers' disease was a problem when women used to make their own gefilte fish. It came from tasting fish before it was thoroughly cooked. It was caused by a parasite in the raw fish.

BE A MR. CLEAN

In the kitchen, think clean.

Poor personal hygiene is another cause of food poisoning. That's why hand washing is so important. "It's particularly important after going to the bathroom," says Schwarz, "because the worst organisms for food-borne illness are fecally transmitted."

The code for institutional food services and restaurants says that you shouldn't smoke while handling food. "The reason has nothing to do with cigarettes," says Schwarz. "It has to do with putting your hand in your mouth. When you smoke, you touch the end of the cigarette, you get saliva on your fingers, and you transmit it to the food. For the same reason, the code requires hand washing after smoking, eating, and drinking." Tasting food can transmit germs, too. To be safe, use a clean spoon each time you taste.

"If you're sick, you probably shouldn't be handling food," cautions Edmund A. Zottola, Ph.D., professor of food microbiology in the Department of Food Science and Nutrition at the University of Minnesota. "The same is true if you have an infected cut, skin irritation, boils, or acne."

KEEP IT SPOTLESS

How clean is clean enough?

Contaminated equipment has been traced to many outbreaks of food-borne disease. It may be obvious that you should use clean utensils when preparing food. But not knowing just what constitutes "clean" has caused many an upset stomach.

After handling raw meat or poultry, always scrub your hands, utensils, and cutting board thoroughly with soap and hot water to prevent cross-contamination. Adding a little chlorine bleach to the rinse helps. Having two cutting boards, one for meat and one for vegetables, can help avoid problems, too. Just make sure the one used for meat gets sanitized, one of the best methods for sanitizing your implements is running them through the dishwasher.

REMEMBER, RAW IS ONLY FOR VEGGIES

"Eating raw meat or seafood is not completely safe," says Patricia Griffin, M.D., an epidemiologist at the Centers for Disease Control. "You're taking a risk. There could be bacteria in them. We strongly advise against drinking raw milk, too. Despite its reputation as a healthy food, raw milk has been the cause of quite a number of outbreaks of food-borne disease because it can carry bacteria. Pasteurization is the best thing that ever happened to milk."

There are risks to eating raw meat and seafood.

In addition, avoid eating raw or soft-boiled eggs, as well as dirty or cracked eggs. The dirt might be chicken manure, teeming with bacteria. But mayonnaise, like most acidic foods, is seldom a cause of food poisoning. It's not until it's mixed with other foods – eggs, tuna, or macaroni, for example – that it becomes a medium for bacterial growth.

Mayonnaise has gotten a bum rap.

You never knew so many miserable germs were hiding in so many unlikely places, did you? Now you do. And now you know how to avoid them.

21

GUILLAIN-BARRÉ SYNDROME: PARALYZED BY A VIRUS

Guillain-Barré is a rare disease that can cause weakness and paralysis.

"The disorder known as Guillain-Barré (ghee-lan bah-ray) syndrome is a rare illness that affects the peripheral nerves of the body," says one of the few nontechnical books written about this mysterious illness. "It can cause weakness and paralysis, as well as abnormal sensations. . . . It can vary greatly in severity, from the mildest case that may not even be brought to a doctor's attention to a devastating illness with almost complete paralysis that brings the patient close to death."

When Diana Tice began developing peculiar symptoms, she had never heard of the disease.

Diana Tice was unaware of that chilling description of Guillain-Barré syndrome (GBS) as she boarded a plane in New York in October 1986. If she had been, she might have paid more attention to the numbness that had mysteriously settled into her hands and feet the previous day. As it was, she hurriedly checked her bags and worried about making her connecting flight to Florida.

Tice did a lot of worrying in those days. An attractive brunette in her thirties, she worked as a marketing representative for one of the largest magazine publishers in the world, selling ad space to clients up and down the East Coast. Much of her working life was a blur of unending hotel rooms, half-eaten dinners, and long evenings spent entertaining corporate ad buyers before boarding another flight the next morning.

"I was feeling tired, miserable, and wretched by the time I reached Florida," she says, "but I was always feeling tired, miserable, and wretched, so I didn't think anything of it."

Tice's condition deteriorated throughout the day, but she went out on her sales call anyway. "I went to see the client and told her I didn't feel well," Tice recalls. "She told me I didn't look very good either and suggested that I stop by an emergency medical center and get checked out."

Her condition deteriorated and medical attention was suggested.

Tice agreed, and it was at the center that she first discovered just how little the medical profession knows about GBS and how hard it can be to diagnose. This is understandable, perhaps, given that no more than 3,000 to 4,000 cases are diagnosed annually. Most physicians will never see a patient with GBS in their entire careers. And, since GBS's early symptoms mimic those of 15 other illnesses (not including mental illness, which is sometimes suspected), it's really not surprising that the doctor at the medical center missed it.

The first doctor she saw failed to diagnose the problem.

"He told me to go back to the hotel and get a good night's sleep," says Tice. "But the next day it was difficult for me to lift my arm to brush my hair. Also, the numbness was moving from my feet to my ankles. I started to get scared and decided to get home as quickly as I could."

Tice called her physician in New York before leaving Florida and told him to expect a visit from her later that day. "Then I put my shoes on and couldn't feel my feet." She arrived back at LaGuardia Airport in the afternoon and hobbled to her car, but once inside discovered she could no longer feel the accelerator or brake pedal. Torn between the possibility of accident and the fear of what was happening inside her body, she switched on the ignition and drove.

Tice drove from the airport without being able to feel her feet.

NERVES UNDER ATTACK

The cause of GBS is unknown. What it does inside the body of its victims is well documented, however, and does much to explain why Diana Tice could not feel her feet that day – or any other part of her body a few days later.

"The body turns on itself," says Guy McKhann, M.D., a neurologist at Johns Hopkins Medical Institute. "Normally, if you're invaded by a foreign antigen, your body makes antibodies against that antigen. Well, in this situation, the patient is making antibodies to his own nerves. The immune system treats the substance that insulates the nerves (myelin) as an antigen and attacks it with antibodies."

In Guillain-Barré, the immune system attacks the substance that coats the nerves.

Why the part of the body responsible for protecting us from harm turns against us this way remains a mystery. No one has explained the attack process on a cellular level. Myelin, for instance, is composed of little more than fats and proteins – why attack that? Yet researchers have noted that a viral attack of one sort or another – a cold, sore throat, stomach, or intestinal illness – sometimes precedes the onset of GBS. Almost as often, however, GBS occurs after seemingly unrelated events, such as an insect bite, surgery, or various injections, such as flu shots.

GBS can occur after an insect bite, surgery, or various injections, but no one knows why.

The most notable injection-related outbreak of GBS took place in the fall of 1976, when millions of Americans were inoculated with the swine flu vaccine. By mid-December, several hundred of those immunized had contracted GBS.

An injection-related outbreak of GBS followed the government's 1976 swine flu vaccination program.

A flurry of damage claims and lawsuits followed. Total paid out by the federal government to date: $91 million. New discoveries made about GBS as a result of this costly, ill-fated vaccination program: one. "The only thing we learned from the swine flu affair is that this disease can occur with vaccines," concedes David Pleasure, M.D., a neurologist at the University of Pennsylvania Hospital.

NUMBNESS, THEN PAIN

One of the first symptoms of a GBS-afflicted body destroying its own nerves is numbness in the feet and hands. Because the attack is carried out 24 hours a day, seven days a week, the numbness usually spreads rapidly once it begins, moving up both sides of the body and into the arms and legs. After that, the nerves controlling the muscles of the arms and legs begin to deteriorate, resulting in great weakness and pain.

It was Saturday afternoon when Diana Tice's illness progressed to that stage. She had made it safely to her doctor's office Friday, but he also failed to recognize GBS in its early stages.

"He told me to go home and come see him on Monday if I still felt bad," Tice recalls. "So I went home and went to sleep." When she woke up the next day, she realized that something was seriously, dreadfully wrong with her. "I felt really bad. The numbness was in my calves, and I had shooting pains up and down my back. I called the doctor and told him he had to do something – today."

Her doctor called the emergency room of the nearest hospital, then told her to meet him there. Finally, in the emergency room, the bits and pieces of Tice's strange illness began adding up. Her doctor mumbled a strange name in what sounded like French. He looked very concerned. Luckily, there was a neurologist on duty in the emergency room. Tice's doctor brought him over to examine her, and the specialist gave his diagnosis. "It's probably Guillain-Barré," he announced. Like most people, Tice had never heard the name before, but she knew it must be serious. "They admitted me to the hospital right then," she says.

A SECOND CHANCE AT LIVING

Kindness? No, a second chance is not always a kindness. Such a thing cannot exist in the

GBS progresses from numbness in the feet and hands to deterioration of nerves controlling the arms and legs.

Her condition was recognized for what it was only after it worsened considerably.

GBS immobilizes its victims, and although it sometimes retreats for a short time, it comes back.

black heart of any disease, and that word should never be applied to GBS. Boredom? Perhaps boredom explains it. If neither of these, then what does account for the behavior of a sickness that, after immobilizing victims so completely that they cannot speak – cannot even breathe – often retreats and leaves them sound again some months later? Why does it stop? Why does GBS give many victims a second chance at life?

Don't ask science. Science can give you the numbers, but not explain the phenomenon. The numbers show that complete recovery is not always the case. Some GBS patients never regain the powers they once had, and up to 5 percent of all its victims die. Another 5 to 15 percent may experience significant long-term disability. Yet 35 percent suffer only mild abnormalities (a lasting numbness in an extremity, perhaps), while more than 50 percent experience complete recovery.

GBS has to run its course; sometimes it kills.

But GBS has a course to run before recovery begins, and that course ends only after a condition known as maximum disability is reached. Maximum disability can mean many things to many people. In some, it may mean nothing more than a brief tingling or weakness in the limbs, typically followed by a sore throat, diarrhea, or other viral symptoms. At its worst, maximum disability can mean almost total paralysis, with severe complications. These include abnormal heartbeat, inability to breathe, massive infections, blood clots, and death.

Diana Tice lay in a New York hospital in a state of maximum disability somewhere between those two extremes. "At its worst, the only part of my body I could move was my head and my right hand," she says. And if the doctors were optimistic about her chances for complete recovery at that point, they weren't saying.

For Tice, severe paralysis lasted a month.

For Tice, severe paralysis lasted a month, though it seemed much longer at the time: "It's a pretty sobering experience when you've been accustomed to doing everything for yourself, and now you need somebody to lift you out of bed and put you on a commode," she says. "It almost got to the point where I had to have someone feed me as well. It was quite a shock."

Yet Tice was lucky in many ways. She lived in a major metropolitan area where sophisticated specialists quickly diagnosed her condition. Now she was undergoing treatment in a modern hospital equipped to handle such cases, under the care of still more specialists.

TREATMENTS OLD AND NEW

Two methods are currently used to treat GBS, and as with many things involving medical specialists, there is debate over which is best.

There is debate over two methods currently used to treat GBS.

The older method is corticosteroid therapy, in which patients are given high doses of the hormone normally made by the adrenal gland. The newer treatment is plasmapheresis, a process in which the plasma is removed from the patient's blood and the red blood cells are pumped back in. Plasmapheresis essentially removes the attacking antibodies from the patient, slowing and easing their assault on the nerves.

"Plasmapheresis is the treatment of choice," says Dr. McKhann, noting that recent studies have shown greatly improved recovery times for GBS patients treated that way. "For most patients, plasmapheresis can shorten recovery by half," he says. "If you do it within two or three days after the disease sets in, recovery is probably quicker than that." What about steroids? "We think there's very little evidence that steroids actually work," he says. But Diana Tice's physicians used steroids, and she did well.

The newer treatment is plasmapheresis, but Tice's physicians used steroids.

Slowly, almost imperceptibly, feeling and strength returned to her body, but she was given precious little time to relax and enjoy the

She was put in physical therapy and her mobility returned.

sensation. "They put me in massive physical therapy," Tice says. "I had to learn how to write again, walk again, do everything again. But that didn't matter – to have my mobility back was all I cared about."

And mobility did return – first with a walker, then with a three-pronged cane, then with a regular cane, and then with no cane at all. "I was back moving and doing things by March," she says, "but it took a full year before I felt 100 percent better. I'm completely recovered now, but I don't know if my chances are better or worse of getting it again. They don't say. I don't think they know."

Tice believes that GBS was her body's way of making her moderate her stressful lifestyle.

In the absence of any data to the contrary, Tice has developed her own theory about Guillain-Barré syndrome, based on first-hand observation: "I believe your mind controls everything that happens to your body," she says. "If I hadn't been traveling constantly, not getting enough sleep, not eating correctly, getting sick all the time, I probably wouldn't have been as prone to getting GBS. Now I try not to run myself ragged or travel as much. I try to lighten up, to have more fun.

"As far as stress or lifestyle bringing GBS on, I'm not sure there's much evidence for that," says Dr. McKhann. "But it could. I mean, there's no question that emotional factors alter the way the immune system functions. So it's conceivable, I suppose."

Even so, "There is nothing you can do that I'm aware of to protect yourself or prevent the onset of this syndrome," he adds. "We just don't know enough about it. I wish I could say there's some major breakthrough in knowledge waiting for us on the horizon. But I'd be exaggerating if I did."

22

HERPES: THE VIRUS THAT ATTACKS YOUR LOVE LIFE

It was time to head for the showers. The aerobics instructor had been a bear, and Amanda, a trim, slim, 50-year-old publishing executive, was dripping with sweat. She headed toward the ladies' locker room. She needed a hot shower, a cold drink, and a place to sit down where the air didn't vibrate with synthesized, amplified, aerobicized rock music.

But those were the three things that Amanda was not going to get. Not after she got a look at the woman sitting on the bench in front of her locker. As the woman smiled a greeting, Amanda saw that her face was marred by the oozing scabs of oral herpes. And as the woman stood up and began to rub her freshly showered body with a towel, Amanda saw the telltale blisters of genital herpes dotting the woman's thighs.

Great. Was the virus on the towel that the woman was now spreading over the bench? Was it on the bench? Could Amanda get it just by sitting down? Could she get it from the shower stall? The drinking fountain? The toilet seat?

Amanda wasn't taking any chances. She smiled at the woman, grabbed her gym bag, and picked up her car keys. The shower, the drink, and the place to sit down could wait until she got home. Home is where more than the heart is, Amanda figured. It's where you find safety and security. It's where you have a fairly good

Can you get herpes from a toilet seat? A shower stall?

idea of what's on the toilet seat besides basin, tub, and tile cleaner.

WHAT YOU CAN CATCH FROM WHERE

Welcome to the 1990s. Where men are men, women are women, and everybody's afraid to sit on the toilet seat. It's the age in which boy-meets-girl pick-up techniques involve a game of Twenty Questions: "Do you know Jerry? How's he doing? Has he recovered from that . . . ah . . . bug he had? Oh, didn't know him that well, huh? Never went out with him? Well . . ."

Welcome to the age in which dentists wear latex gloves, kissin' cousins don't kiss, and the only "safe sex" is no sex, married sex, or virgin sex. Welcome to the age of herpes.

Once you get oral or genital herpes, it is with you forever.

Herpes is a family of viruses in which one single brother/sister act – oral herpes and genital herpes – has terrorized the United States more effectively than the PLO. Both are characterized by painful blisters that ooze – on and around your mouth in oral herpes, on and around your genitals, buttocks, and anus in genital herpes. Both are with you forever. Even if you never have a second outbreak of either, the virus hides away in a nerve, waiting for the proper combination of stress, exhaustion, menstruation, poor nutrition, food sensitivity (especially to arginine-rich foods such as turkey, nuts, eggs, milk, and cheese), emotional upset, even sunburn to pop out and display itself on your face and/or bottom. It's almost as though anything that suppresses or upsets your immune system can reactivate the virus.

About 70 percent of us first get oral herpes in infancy or early childhood, doctors say. Children infected with the virus may have an inflammation of the throat or gums, fever, blisters in the mouth or throat (sometimes called fever blisters or cold sores), mouth pain, or no symptoms at all.

Where does the virus come from? At least 17 percent of infantile herpes comes from a parent, grandparent, or loving caregiver who has a cold sore, says Lisa M. Frenkel, M.D., an assistant professor of pediatrics at UCLA. The adult either kisses the child or inadvertently touches their own mouth and then the child.

Genital herpes is just as infectious, although it frequently limits itself to a single, nasty episode. While some adults may have gotten it at birth from an infected mother, most contract the virus as a result of close body contact – kissing, intercourse, oral or anal sex. Initially, doctors thought that someone would have to have oozing blisters before the virus could be transmitted, but recent studies have indicated that you can get the virus from someone who has absolutely no sign of it. And condoms and spermicides – although they are recommended by doctors – protect only the area they cover.

Genital herpes usually comes from close body contact.

Researchers *have* found that the virus can also live on inanimate objects such as a plastic toilet seat for 1½ hours. But retrieving a specimen of herpes from a toilet seat in the lab and actually being infected by it when you sit down in a public rest room are two different things, explains Sandra Schwarcz, M.D., a staff physician at the Centers for Disease Control.

Herpes virus *can* live on a toilet seat, but catching it that way is unlikely.

The difference, says Jerrold J. Ellner, M.D., professor of medicine at Case Western Reserve University School of Medicine and director of infectious diseases at Cleveland's University Hospitals, may be a question of intensity. "It may be that a certain intensity of exposure is necessary," he says, "one that you can get from close personal contact but that you can't get from a toilet seat."

PREVENTING FLARE-UPS

Herpes can't be cured, but it can be treated.

Fortunately, although herpes cannot be cured, it can be treated to minimize symptoms and recurrence. The treatment of choice, doctors say, is acyclovir, administered orally, topically – or should you have a complication such as meningitis – intravenously in the hospital. Topical acyclovir is frequently used to decrease the size and severity of oral herpes sores, while acyclovir in pill form is used both as a treatment and as a daily prophylactic to prevent flare-ups of genital herpes. When acyclovir does not prevent recurrences of genital herpes, a study conducted by a team of researchers at UCLA indicates that interferon may do the job.

The UCLA team organized 76 people who had eight or more recurrences of genital herpes a year into two groups. One group received either a fake pill or a low, ineffective dose of interferon three times a week for 12 weeks. The other group received a much higher dose of interferon in the same manner. The result? The higher-dose group had fewer outbreaks during the study, a shorter period of active infection, less itching, and faster healing. And the time between flare-ups was *doubled*.

Supplements of the amino acid lysine and stress reduction can help.

Another strategy to prevent recurrence of both oral and genital herpes may be supplements of the amino acid lysine. The idea is still controversial – which means you should check with your doctor before you try it yourself – but in a recent study at the Indiana University School of Medicine, 27 people with recurrent oral herpes, genital herpes, or both took 3 grams of lysine daily for six months. They reported significantly less severe symptoms, faster healing, and half the recurrences they'd expected.

How did the lysine work? The researchers think that lysine competes with another amino acid, arginine, for your body's attention. When your body pays attention to the lysine, it doesn't interact with the arginine, an element that's essential for replication of the herpes virus. No arginine, no herpes. Or certainly less of it.

A third strategy to prevent the recurrence of herpes may be relaxation. "Stress clearly leads to recurrences of oral herpes," says Dr. Ellner. "Its role in genital herpes is much less clear, but we do find that the higher the stress, the more lab evidence of immunosuppression." And a suppressed immune system, he adds, is what allows the virus to break out of hiding and erupt in sores.

How does stress work? Dr. Ellner speculates that beta-endorphins, which are chemicals released by your body in response to stress, activate suppressor T-cells in people who have frequent recurrences. Dr. Ellner's research suggests that the suppressor cells then interfere with two critical antiviral mechanisms: interleukin-2, which is needed by your body to produce activated T-cells, and natural killer cells, which are the immune system commandos that are charged with hunting down a virus-infected cell and zapping it into oblivion.

"Fortunately, many people have only a single episode of herpes," says Dr. Ellner. But when they have frequent recurrences, a stress-reduction program may be the answer. There is some evidence that learning how to modify the way you react to a stressful event – a poor performance rating from your boss, divorce papers from your husband, a lab slip that confirms the diagnosis of herpes – can modify your immune system. And that, suggests Dr. Ellner, may also decrease your body's susceptibility to a flare-up.

Learning how to deal with stress may help control herpes flare-ups.

23

IMAGERY: TALKING TO YOUR IMMUNE SYSTEM

Imagine you're dining at the Café des Artistes in New York. You've just finished $100 worth of broccoli bisque, smoked salmon, and sautéed scallops. And now you're ready for dessert. Your waiter suggests you glance toward the heavy oak dessert cart – just to your left – and see what tempts your taste buds.

Images of delicious food can stimulate your salivary glands.

Mmmmmm. The cart is an island, sparkling amid the sophisticated diners who surround it. Mounds of pure, white ice are studded with strawberries, raspberries, and blueberries, with a bowl of creamy lemon soufflé in the center. A glass shelf floating above the buffet features a buttery confection of apples, walnuts, and cinnamon at one end, an orgy of cream and oranges whipped together at the other. And in the center rises a rich chocolate torte, smothered in mocha buttercream, studded with walnuts, crowned with a dollop of whipped cream that simply overwhelms the senses. You can just taste the rich, smooth, velvety chocolate, can't you?

SPEAK YOUR BODY'S LANGUAGE

If you're starting to salivate, it's your own fault. It's your own fault because you just spoke to your salivary glands in a language they understand. The image of chocolate was translated by

174

your brain into patterns that told those glands to prepare for action. And if you held the image long enough, your stomach probably started to contract.

"Imagery is the way we send messages to our body," explains Errol R. Korn, M.D., a clinical associate at the University of California, San Diego. "It sends messages to the deeper parts of the brain, and the brain then translates those messages into action. It's one of the ways – if not the only practical way – to get into the unconscious mind."

Imagery is a way to talk to your body.

In the first scientific attempt to document the effects of imagery on the body, for example, a 39-year-old woman participated in a study at the University of Arkansas in which she used imagery to manipulate her reaction to an injection of the virus that causes chickenpox.

One woman uses a healing image.

The first step of the study was to find out her normal reaction to chickenpox, especially since she'd already had the disease. So the researchers injected her arm with the virus, then waited for her immune system's reaction. And within 48 hours, a small, nickel-size blister had appeared, as did a slight increase in the activity of her white blood cells as they mustered to fight the invader.

The researchers repeated the test, and the woman responded with a second blister and a second increase in white blood cells. Then the researchers suggested that the woman, who usually practiced a relaxation exercise twice daily for 30 minutes at a time, try to reduce the blister during the next test by adding 5 minutes of imagery to her relaxation exercise.

The woman did. After cautioning her body not to do anything that would leave her open to infection, she began to visualize the blister on her arm getting smaller and smaller. Then, after the next injection of virus, she passed her hand over her arm, sending an imagined "healing energy" to the injection site.

The results were amazing. Not only was this blister significantly smaller than the preceding ones, but a laboratory analysis of the woman's white blood cells revealed that their activity level had plummeted!

TURN YOUR IMMUNE SYSTEM UP

Of course, most of us aren't trying to turn our immune system down. We're trying to turn it up. But does having the ability to turn your immune system down mean you also have the ability to turn it up? Can you actually use imagery to boost your body's resistance?

Yes, says Martin L. Rossman, M.D., a clinical associate at the University of California, San Francisco, you can. And you may also be able to use imagery to find out why your immune system isn't working up to par.

Your body just may talk back.

An inward scanning of your body frequently reveals problems, because imagery is a two-way street. "It's a language of communication between body and mind. If you take some time to learn how it works, your body can use it to send you messages about what's wrong. And then you can solve problems or send positive messages back to make it function better," he explains.

One of his patients, who was plagued with allergies, imaged a master controller of his immune system, says Dr. Rossman. The controller was exhausted, draped over a desk in a control room filled with TV screens and computers.

The man talked with the master controller and asked him what he needed. The controller pointed toward a ball dimly glowing in the middle of the room – a power source that he said was fading. The man walked over to the ball, empathized – "I know how you feel" – then touched the ball and allowed it to feel his concern. And the more he communicated with the ball, the stronger the controller got.

Finally he asked what he could do to give the ball even more energy, and the answer that came back, says Dr. Rossman, was the need for certain nutrients and some emotional support. He got both, he says, presumably giving his exhausted immune system a boost. In any case, his allergies ceased to disrupt his life. He had talked to his immune system in its language of images and it had replied.

SEND A HEALING IMAGE

So how would you like to pull up a chair and have a talk with your immune system? Go ahead, urges Dr. Rossman. And if you suspect there's an illness, make an appointment with your doctor to check it out, and then think about sending your immune system a healing image.

"For relatively minor illnesses like hay fever, doing relaxation and imagery exercises for 15 or 20 minutes twice a day may give you some relief," says Dr. Rossman. "For seriously ill people with diseases like cancer, however, the people who get the best results do it 2 or 3 hours a day."

Twenty-minute imagery exercises twice a day may help.

Between imaging sessions, be careful not to worry about your illness. Worry is a kind of uncontrolled imagery that can negatively affect your health, cautions Dr. Rossman. If you constantly have worst-case scenarios running through your head, you may literally be telling your body to carry them out.

Worry is a kind of uncontrolled imagery that can negatively affect your health.

Ready for some healthy imaging? Begin with a relaxation exercise and then use this image, developed by Dr. Korn, to tell your immune

Here's an image of light.

system what you expect. You might even want to put the exercise on tape and then play it back after you've entered a state of deep relaxation.

Allow yourself to concentrate . . . on an area in the midportion of your forehead . . . so that you may even begin to feel . . . a tingling sensation. . . . As you do so . . . you are bringing all your attention . . . all your consciousness . . . to this area. . . . By centering your consciousness . . . you can bring the . . . full power . . . of it to . . . enhance . . . the establishment of . . . wellness . . . in the body/mind axis. . . . Now allow the spot of attention . . . to become as small as you possibly can . . . so that all your consciousness is . . . concentrated . . . in a very small area. . . . Now project this point . . . to an area about a foot above your head . . . and let it expand . . . to the size of a baseball. . . . Let this sphere obtain the appearance of . . . a glowing sphere . . . of radiant . . . fiery . . . white . . . light. . . . Perceive the glowing and fiery nature . . . feel the warmth . . . and maybe even hear . . . the vibratory qualities of this object. . . . Now let it begin to slowly . . . expand . . . until it achieves the size of a moderately sized melon . . . still radiant . . . fiery . . . glowing . . . white. . . . Allow the bottom to open . . . as though the top were hinged . . . and as it does . . . begin to see the downpour of fiery . . . white . . . radiant . . . light energy. . . . Feel and see the energy entering the body through the top of the head . . . and flowing downward through the entire body . . . from the head . . . into the neck . . . down the arms to the hands . . . back up the arms . . . down the chest . . . both front and back . . . the remainder of the trunk . . . front and back . . . down into the legs . . . the feet . . . and out the feet . . . into the ground. . . . Permit yourself not only to see the energy pour through the body . . . but feel it . . . and also hear it. . . . True health and wellness will be exemplified by a . . . free flow . . . of this fiery . . . radiant . . . white

... light ... energy through the body. ... If there are problems in the body such as diseases or discomforts ... whether they be consciously realized or not ... they can be manifested by some weakness ... or even a complete blockage ... of the flow of this fiery ... radiant ... white ... light ... energy ... through that particular area or areas of the body. ... When these areas are perceived ... you may be able to feel and see these areas being fragmented ... and consumed ... by this fiery ... radiant ... white ... light ... energy. ... It is as though the debris and garbage of the body ... were being incinerated ... by this ... healing force. ... When the discomfort ... disorder ... or diseases have been fragmented and consumed ... by this fiery ... radiant ... white ... light ... energy ... the result will be ... free flow ... of energy ... through this area. ... Continue to feel ... and perceive ... through this downpour ... coming from that sphere ... above the head through the entire body ... and out the feet ... and into the floor ... until the free flow ... of this fiery ... radiant ... white ... light ... energy ... has been established through the body ... so when this free flow has been established ... it will represent the elimination of all toxins ... wastes ... and debris ... that interfere with the ... maintenance of health. ... When this free flow has been established ... allow the sphere to close ... and the downpour to cease. ... Then allow the sphere ... to get larger ... approximately 3 feet in diameter ... and allow it to rotate ... very slowly ... around its vertical axis. ... As it rotates ... allow it to descend ... very slowly ... so that it descends ... around the entire body ... from head ... to toes. ... The function of the sphere at this time ... is to absorb any accumulated debris ... that has been left behind by the radiant ... light ... downpour. ... When it reaches the feet ... the entire body should be cleansed of all debris ... detrimental to maintenance of physical . . . and emotional . . . wellness. . . . Now let the sphere begin to . . . slowly . . . rotate . . . in the opposite direction . . . around its vertical axis . . . and let it slowly begin to ascend . . . the body. . . . The function . . . of the sphere . . . at this time is to . . . instill . . . new . . . and vitalizing . . . energy . . . into the body. . . . Not only is the energy being instilled into the body . . . but it is being instilled . . . into a body . . . which has been completely freed . . . of all forces which would hinder the . . . complete assimilation and utilization . . . of this energy. . . . When the sphere reaches the top of the head . . . then ascends . . . above the head . . . the entire . . . body/mind axis . . . can be free . . . of all debris . . . and filled with a vitality . . . and energy . . . heretofore rarely if ever experienced. . . . The sphere can now . . . stop rotating . . . and begin to . . . shrink . . . in size and eventually . . . return to the body as a point of . . . concentrated consciousness . . . in the forehead region. . . . Then, with a few deep breaths . . . this consciousness can travel throughout the body . . . and you can return slowly to the waking state.

Peace.

24

INFLAMMATORY BOWEL DISEASE: THE GUT UNDER FIRE

Max Brown stood by the barbecue grill, turning steaks, dodging smoke, slapping mosquitoes, and cracking jokes. All that manic activity couldn't hide the dark circles under his eyes, the way he seemed to catch his breath between words, or the way his clothes – a collared sport shirt and a pair of khaki slacks – seemed to hang away from his body. Nor did it hide the way his body itself seemed to hang, suspended, over the grill as though all 6 feet of him were about to topple over.

But the guests at this backyard bash never said a word about their host's obvious exhaustion. They knew he had ulcerative colitis, a chronic inflammatory bowel disease (IBD) in which intestinal spasms twist your gut with pain and "Where's the bathroom?" becomes the most – the only – important question in life. And they knew that Max's determination to ignore the disease and live a normal life would keep him turning out perfectly cooked, medium-rare steaks until every last aunt, uncle, niece, and in-law was stuffed full of USDA prime.

Max is that kind of guy.

"Where's the bathroom?" becomes the most important question in life.

A FLOOD
OF IMMUNE SYSTEM PLAYERS

Until recently, there wasn't much medical science could tell someone like Max about IBD. Doctors could tell him that the disease generally appeared as an inflammation of either the large intestine or rectum – in which case it's called ulcerative colitis – or as an inflammation of the small intestine – usually referred to as Crohn's disease.

They could tell him that the symptoms of IBD – the inflammation, the swelling, the diarrhea, and the constant feeling of having to defecate – were all caused by a flood of immune system players. Where these defensive players came from and who called them in is anybody's guess. A rogue gene from Max's mom or dad, a defect in his immune system, an allergen that plays hide and seek right through the walls of his intestine, or a bacterium that hit him with an infection, set up an inflammatory response, then departed for parts unknown are all under suspicion.

Unfortunately, once the immune system initiates this kind of inflammatory response, it can become almost self-perpetuating no matter what the cause. IBD is a disease that smolders even when it's in remission.

It's almost as though your gut has been bombed by an old B-52.

"Once there's damage to the gut," explains gastroenterologist Richard P. MacDermott, M.D., associate professor of medicine at Washington University Medical School in St. Louis, "then a lot of things can [aggravate it] because all the barriers are lost." It's almost as though your gut has been bombed by an old B-52. And wherever there's now a break in the lining of your gut, bacteria and even the peppers from last night's pizza can slip through and stir up the embers of inflammation.

PUTTING OUT THE FIRE

That's why doctors frequently advise a diet of clear liquids during an attack of IBD, says Dr. MacDermott. Fat-free broths, bouillons, clear fruit juices that have been diluted with water, Kool-Aid, Popsicles, gelatin, and carbonated beverages without caffeine can prevent dehydration while your doctor tries to smother the inflammation with a fusillade of drugs such as corticosteroid immunosuppressives.

Clear liquids can calm your digestive tract.

Unfortunately, malnutrition is frequently a side effect of this kind of treatment. It can be caused by an interaction between nutrients and the drugs you're taking to reduce the inflammation.

Malnutrition is frequently a side effect.

Corticosteroids, for example, can decrease your absorption of calcium and phosphorus while they increase urinary losses of vitamin C, calcium, potassium, and zinc. Sulfasalazine, a mainstay of IBD treatment, interferes with folate absorption. And cholestyramine interferes with the absorption of vitamins A, B_{12}, D, E, and K, as well as folate, calcium, and iron.

AVOIDING MALNUTRITION

How can you avoid malnutrition? Even if you're on a clear liquid diet, you can still choose to buy Popsicles made out of fruit juices rather than the commercial brands made out of sugar, water, and artificial coloring. And when IBD is active, some doctors prescribe special liquids that are a concentrated form of food.

Moreover, when the disease relaxes its hold on your gut even temporarily, you can restock your nutrient stores by eating a wide variety of foods rich in the nutrients that your particular drug/diet regimen may affect.

Restock your nutrient stores when the disease relaxes its hold.

Not that eating is always easy. Fortunately, you may find that frequent, small meals are less likely to cause intestinal cramping than three squares a day. And an antispasmodic drug, prescribed by your doctor and taken 15 or 20 minutes before eating, may help you sit through a meal without having to run to the bathroom.

Avoiding foods high in fiber and fat may also be helpful, as will avoiding any particular food that seems to trigger cramping. And if you're one of the rare individuals with low levels of an enzyme called lactase, either avoiding dairy products or adding a lactase supplement to milk may prevent further aggravation of your disease. These supplements are available at drugstores.

A NEW DISCOVERY

Nearly one-third of those with IBD are addicted to painkillers.

Although diet, drugs, and even surgery relieve the active symptoms of IBD to some degree, somewhere between 15 and 75 percent of those who are afflicted will experience one relapse after another, and their lives will be constantly distorted by fear: fear of embarrassing accidents, fear of an increased incidence of cancer, and fear of drug dependency. The incidence of addiction to painkillers, for example, ranges around 30 percent in those with IBD.

It's not a pleasant life. But a new discovery from a curious group of stress researchers at UCLA and the Harvard Medical School may soon prevent relapses and, for all intents and purposes, provide a cure for the disease.

Stress frequently precipitates an attack of IBD.

How did stress researchers end up studying IBD? "We knew that stress was involved in flare-ups and often actually precipitated inflammatory bowel disease," says Patrick Mantyh, Ph.D., an assistant professor of medicine at UCLA. "The question was: 'How does it do that?' " After all, the brain must translate stress into a chemical

language the body understands and then somehow communicate it to the gut.

"What were the neurotransmitters used to
communicate that information?" asks Dr. Mantyh.
"And how did they do it?"

The researchers looked around for something they could use as a model to guide their
thinking. "One [example] that was suggestive of
what might be going on was the herpes virus,"
recalls Dr. Mantyh. "The virus is usually taken up
on the skin and is harbored in the sensory nerves –
the nerves that more or less form the bridge
between the skin and the brain.

Nerves form a bridge between the skin and the brain.

"Most [scientists] thought the nerves' sole
function was to sense what happens out in the
peripheral tissue – the skin – and communicate
that to the brain. But we thought that this might
really be a two-way street – that the brain could
also tell that sensory neuron what to do out in
the skin.

"So we focused on that neuron and said,
'Well, we know that in the last five years or so
people have described several neurotransmitters that are present in these sensory neurons –
small neuropeptides [such as substance P] that
are thought to be involved in mediating pain.'
Then we said, 'All right, we know who these
neurotransmitters are, let's see where they actually have an action out in the skin, or in this case,
in the inflammatory bowel tissue.'"

The researchers set to work. They obtained
surgical samples of bowel tissue from people
with and without IBD and examined it under
their microscopes. But how could they tell if the
neurotransmitters were actually affecting the
bowel?

"When a sensory neuron releases a neurotransmitter," explains Dr. Mantyh, "it interacts
with something on the target tissue. That something's called a receptor. They fit together like a
lock and key, with the key being the neurotrans-

The researchers put a radio-active tag on the neurotrans-mitter and watched where it went.

mitter, the lock being the receptor." To figure out where the neurotransmitter was going, says Dr. Mantyh, the researchers put a radioactive tag on the neurotransmitter and watched where it went.

"It was a startling finding," acknowledges Dr. Mantyh. The blood vessels and immune system cells in tissue taken from people with IBD was covered with more than *2,000* receptors. The tissue taken from people without IBD had none – absolutely zero.

It makes a beeline for receptors on the immune system cells in your gut—and the by-product is pain.

That's why stress can trigger an attack of pain, swelling, and diarrhea in those with IBD, explains Dr. Mantyh. Stress causes the sensory neuron to generate a neurotransmitter called substance P, which then makes a beeline for its receptors on the immune system cells in your gut. The cells respond as good immune system cells always respond to an attack – with a flood of defensive plays and lots of inflammation. Pain is an unfortunate by-product of the process.

THE CURE

Now that scientists know how the inflammatory process is triggered in those with IBD, a solution is at hand. "What we're now trying to do is get something to block that receptor – to antagonize that [inflammatory] response," says Dr. Mantyh.

And it won't take another ten years of mucking about in the lab. "In the last two or three years, two groups [of researchers] have been successful in being able to make stable antagonists to neuropeptides other than substance P. I think that more or less gives us a model of how to go about it. So we're using that same technique to develop the one for substance P."

A cure for Max.

How long until he finds the antagonist that will prevent the fire of IBD? He'll probably have it by the time Max Brown flips his next steak.

25

INFLUENZA:
LAST OF THE GREAT PLAGUES

It begins with a shiver, a cough, an ache. Your temperature climbs above a hundred and your reaction time is reduced by half. It's not a cold – colds include a sore throat and a runny nose, but no fever, ache, or slow reactions – and it's not measles, mumps, or rubella. They, you'll recall, have spots.

So what is it that leaves you feeling like the victim of a hit and run? It's the flu – also known as the bug, the grippe, or influenza – and when it hits, says Edwin D. Kilbourne, M.D., chairman of the Microbiology Department at Mount Sinai School of Medicine in New York, it knocks you off your feet and into your bed.

When the flu hits, it knocks you off your feet and into your bed.

It's caused by a virus lodged smack in the middle of your respiratory system – nobody knows why the aches and pains travel when the virus doesn't – and it's probably been incubating there for two or three days before you developed any symptoms. You can also count on it hanging around for three to six days more.

But influenza is more than an annoyance that costs you a few days of work or pleasure, says Dr. Kilbourne. Influenza can kill. It sets up housekeeping in a cell and breeds faster than a hutch of rabbits while it plays hide and seek with your immune system. And until the good guys overcome the bad guys at the cellular level, there's not a lot that you can do except avoid

Caused by a virus, influenza can kill.

driving – influenza slows your reaction time – and take it easy.

Amantadine, an antiviral drug, might reduce the length of your illness from three or four days to one or two, says Dr. Kilbourne, but it's still a case of the flu. That's why amantadine, which can also be used to prevent the flu on a short-term basis, is usually reserved for preventing the development of new cases among groups of high-risk people – those over age 65 who may have hidden heart or lung problems – who have not already been immunized. (Amantadine takes effect quickly, while a regular vaccine takes nine or ten days.)

If flu develops, it's particularly important that those with heart problems take it easy. A small spot of inflammation can develop on the heart. If you refuse to slow down, the inflammation can spread and lead to heart failure or irregular heart rhythms.

GETTING OFF LIGHTLY

If influenza lets you off lightly, you're one of the lucky ones.

But just as high-risk people are more likely to get a bad case of flu, says Dr. Kilbourne, other people are more likely to get off lightly. And when these lucky folks take a shortcut through the illness, it's usually because their immune system simply has more experience handling the virus.

How do you get to be an experienced virus handler? "The entire population is a mosaic of virus experience," says Dr. Kilbourne. A virus comes through, you get it, your body develops antibodies that shoot it down and posts a "no admittance" sign in its memory banks.

But the virus can't survive or reproduce without a nice warm human to call home. So in its desperation to be readmitted to your body, it has developed the incredible ability to change its clothes – to literally change its surface –

enabling it to hide from your immune system. When it knocks on your respiratory door a second time, it's disguised enough so that your immune system lets it in. Your immune system won't be fooled for very long – that's why you won't get as sick as someone who's never had it – but you still won't feel very well for a couple of days.

The fact that an influenza virus has this chameleonlike ability explains why making an effective vaccine is so difficult. "We're always playing catch-up," says Dr. Kilbourne. "The best we can do is to watch [the current virus] around the globe, particularly where it's south of the equator. As new viruses appear, we make educated guesses as to what strains should be included in the next flu vaccine, and then we try to grow them."

Because the composition of a vaccine is changed as new viruses develop, it's important to get a flu shot every year. An updated vaccine manages to keep 80 percent of the people who get it pretty healthy.

New vaccines are required each year to fight flu viruses.

Unfortunately, the vaccine has not been very effective with either the oldest or the youngest in our society. In a study at UCLA, for example, flu shots protected less than 10 percent of the 87 residents in a nursing home where flu was epidemic. It did, however, mean a milder case for some, and a review of studies subsequently conducted by the researchers indicates that the shots can reduce the risk of death associated with influenza by as much as 75 percent.

Flu shots frequently don't work in older people.

DRUGS DISABLE THE VACCINE

Part of the reason flu shots frequently don't work in older people, says Charles John Schleupner, M.D., head of infectious diseases at Salem Veterans Administration Medical Center and an associate professor of medicine at the

University of Virginia, is that older folks are frequently taking regular medication such as aspirin or calcium channel blockers – frequently prescribed for heart problems – that suppress their immune response to the vaccine. Another reason may be the fact that the immune systems of adults over 65 are simply not that efficient.

Scientists are working on new flu vaccines.

But scientists may have figured out a strategy to overcome the problem, says Dr. Schleupner. They've developed a new vaccine for influenza by hooking the old vaccine up with a diphtheria toxoid – a protein derived from the bacteria that cause diphtheria – to give the immune system a larger target. A larger target, they hope, will mean a larger response. And that means better protection.

Using this kind of strategy, scientists are now developing various vaccines for both children under 1 year and adults over 65. The vaccine for older folks has just moved out of the lab and into human testing. If all goes well, all of us – young and old alike – should soon be protected from what doctors call the last great plague.

26

INTERFERON:
THE MAGIC BULLET RICOCHETS

Interferon was greeted with hosannas. The cry went up from suffering humanity in the 1960s and grew even louder in the 1970s. The chemical discovered hidden within the human body in minute quantities was *it*. The panacea of the 20th century. The mythological magic bullet that was going to shoot down the cancer monster, punch a hole in multiple sclerosis, fell humanity's worst viral infections like so many cardboard ducks.

"People wanted it in their hands, in their body, within days when they heard it could be produced in large quantities," says Thomas Merigan, M.D., professor of medicine and head of the Division of Infectious Diseases at Stanford University School of Medicine.

So, whatever happened to interferon?

The interferon magic bullet was fired all right. Many times. It ricocheted off the public's extravagant enthusiasm and plowed right into scientific reality.

"*Nothing* is the magic bullet. That's the issue," says Dr. Merigan. "Everything has certain unique applications, and it takes money and time to find those."

THE MYSTERY UNFOLDS ... SLOWLY

Discovered in 1957, interferon is one of a number of chemical messengers that the immune

Interferon once generated a lot of enthusiasm. Where is it now?

Researchers have experimented with interferon since 1957.

191

Initially interferon showed incredible promise, but it was in very short supply.

system uses to communicate. The immune system uses chemicals almost like a telephone, calling up whole armies of fighter cells and sending them into battle. When scientists first started experimenting with interferon, some people thought they had captured the Ma Bell of the human immune system. They couldn't wait to start sending coded messages of their own: "Get to work!" "Zap that cancer!" "Smash that virus!"

In early experiments in test tubes and with animals, interferon showed incredible promise as a cancer-fighting agent. Scientists got excited. Journalists got excited. People reading about it, especially sick people, got *really* excited.

At first it was hard for scientists to get enough of the stuff to experiment with.

"Interferon can be made in human white blood cells, but in infinitesimally small quantities. It was very laborious, very expensive, and very difficult to make enough of it," says Jan Vilcek, M.D., Ph.D, professor of microbiology at New York University Medical Center.

It took almost 20 years for scientists to learn how to purify interferon and to create the technology to produce it in sufficient quantities to conduct the necessary research. Human interferon is now produced through genetic engineering technology.

It became available in larger quantities and was found to have limitations.

When scientists finally got to test interferon on large numbers of people, they found what many of them had suspected all along – that interferon was not going to be a cancer cure-all. Or any other kind of a cure-all.

"We learn in man that there are always unexpected problems in the application. And you can't count your chickens before they're hatched," says Dr. Merigan.

THERE'S MORE TO COME

Interferon is used to treat some cancers, hepatitis, and genital warts.

Interferon didn't fail. It just didn't live up to expectations. While there are a number of cancers that interferon won't touch, it is now licensed for use as a therapeutic agent for hairy cell leukemia, a rare form of cancer.

In Japan, interferon is being used against some forms of hepatitis. And in this country, it is being studied as a nasal spray to prevent the common cold and as an antiwart drug. Interferon seems to be very good against genital warts, says Dr. Merigan.

The research goes on. Scientists are still learning about what the various types of interferon (there are several) do in the body.

"To be perfectly honest, the complete functions of interferon in the body are not understood," says Dr. Vilcek. "It is important in the regulation of antibody synthesis. It is important in the regulation of some specialized forms of human white blood cells that will engulf and destroy various infectious agents and also act as helper T-cells in the production of antibodies."

Dr. Merigan continues to study interferon's use in combination with other drugs. He expects that in the future interferon will prove useful against several other forms of cancer and some viral infections, including the AIDS virus.

Dr. Vilcek is studying some of the other chemical messengers of the immune system, including interleukins and tumor necrosis factor (TNF). Perhaps these substances that are produced by the human body will someday yield other useful drugs in the ongoing fight against cancer and infection.

Other chemical messengers of the immune system are now being studied.

"I would certainly hope so," says Dr. Vilcek. "But I wouldn't want to repeat the mistake that was made with interferon and come up with unrealistic predictions and expectations."

Amen.

27

KIDNEY DISEASE: AN IMMUNE SYSTEM MALFUNCTION

An epidemic occurs in the Zuni Indian population.

The Zuni Indians are dying. High in the mountains of western New Mexico, in a pueblo where women still bake the day's bread in clay ovens outside their homes, the Zuni are succumbing to an epidemic of kidney disease at a rate 14 times higher than that of their white neighbors.

Nobody is sure of the cause, says Donald M. Megill, M.D., an Indian Public Health Service kidney specialist who has studied the Indians. But most of the disease, he suspects, is triggered by the Zuni's immune system.

How? "There are two major ways in which the immune system can injure the kidney," explains Peter M. Burkholder, M.D., a professor of pathology at the University of Michigan Medical School, who has studied kidney problems. "The formation of circulating immune complexes – leftover pieces of antibodies and the invaders they destroyed during an infection – is one. And the formation of auto-antibodies – antibodies that attack what they're supposed to defend – is another," he explains. These can develop in all of us, not just Zuni Indians.

Kidney disease can be caused by leftover debris after you've had pneumonia or strep.

Immune complexes are normally formed after an infection such as pneumonia, strep, or staph, says Dr. Burkholder. They're battlefield garbage that is picked up in your bloodstream

194

and sent to the kidneys. There your body sorts debris into what can be recycled and what should be thrown out. The material that can be recycled – water, for example – is sent back into your bloodstream for reuse. The remainder that your body can't use – urea, trace metals, amino acids – is sent to the bladder for elimination.

But, for some reason scientists don't understand, says Dr. Burkholder, immune complexes – which are supposed to be on their way to your bladder – sometimes get stuck in your kidney. And that kind of molecular roadblock activates your immune system all over again. Neutrophils – those hungry scavengers that swallow bacteria and then dissolve them in toxic enzymes – rush to the rescue. They invade your kidney, surround the immune complexes and the tissue in which they're stuck, and – in an effort to "save you" – secrete enzymes that eat your kidney.

"The kidney's like an innocent bystander that got hit," says Dr. Burkholder. In rapidly progressing kidney disease, the result is as though a hand grenade had gone off. Your kidney is punched full of holes and its contents dumped into your urine.

"The kidney's like an innocent bystander that got hit," says one scientist.

The result of an attack by auto-antibodies is much the same. Auto-antibodies don't circulate through the blood the way immune complexes do, says Dr. Burkholder. Instead they target a particular organ – the kidney, in this instance – as an enemy invader and launch a full-scale attack.

Why? Well, one theory is that something your immune system perceives as an invader has been deposited in your kidney. And the antibody is really targeting the invader. After a bout of viral pneumonia, for example, a partially destroyed virus may be traveling through the kidney on its way out of your body. Somehow your immune system identifies it as a threat, stimulates the production of antibodies, and attacks your kidney along with the virus. Again, your kidney is just an innocent bystander.

HELPING YOUR KIDNEY FIGHT BACK

Your kidney is a regenerative champ.

Somewhere between 85 and 90 percent of all kidney disease in humans is caused by an immune response of one sort or another, says Dr. Burkholder. Fortunately, your kidney has marvelous regenerative capabilities.

"Kidney disease is not a death sentence," emphasizes Richard J. Glassock, M.D., who chairs the Department of Medicine at the Harbor-UCLA Medical Center. More than half of all kidney disease triggered by your immune system does not progress to renal failure – the point at which you can die because your kidneys can't do their job. Half does progress, but it's a process that can take up to 30 or 40 years.

"You can help some people very dramatically by providing drugs – chemical agents that affect the antibody-producing cells," says Dr. Glassock. "Or you can remove antibodies from the patient's blood by plasma exchange," a process in which a machine literally sifts auto-antibodies out of your blood.

A diet rich in fish oils may be able to slow the disease.

But a primary tactic to delay the onset of renal failure is diet. There's evidence – primarily in the lab – that a diet rich in omega-3 fatty acids from fish oils can suppress the number of hand grenades thrown at your kidneys by an immune system on the attack.

A special diet can protect the kidneys from damage.

"And for any form of kidney disease that does progress to kidney failure, there's evidence – lots in the lab, some in man – that a low-protein, low-calorie, low-phosphorus, and low-salt diet will slow the rate of failure," he says.

How does he translate "low?" "Low-protein means something on the order of 40 grams of protein per day," says Dr. Glassock, which – for most of us – means cutting daily consumption by about a third. Fortunately, in most cases, cutting protein by that much will also cut calories.

And phosphorus, which is found primarily in dairy products, should not exceed 750 milligrams per day – roughly 3 cups of milk. Salt consumption should also be reduced to 4 or 5 grams a day, says Dr. Glassock, including the hidden salt found in lunch meats and packaged cereals.

This diet is effective only when there's impairment of kidney function, cautions Dr. Glassock. "The best evidence to date is that it modifies the renal circulation to lower pressure within the kidney's capillaries. That protects the kidney from damage," and, as other scientists have recently discovered, it also seems to reduce the number of immune complexes that get stuck in the kidney.

That's good news, of course, particularly for the Zuni Indians. Because a genetic predisposition to developing immune complexes, says the Indian Public Health Service's Dr. Megill, seems to be what's causing the Zuni epidemic.

The diet also reduces the number of immune complexes that get stuck in the kidney.

28

LEFT-HANDEDNESS: AUTOIMMUNITY'S SOUTHPAWS

It's a right-handed world.

Left-handed people make better bowlers. (They tend to use the smoother left side of the bowling lane.) And they make better typists. (The most-used keys are on the left side of the keyboard.) Southpaw tennis players, boxers, and baseball players have an advantage over right-handed opponents who have to adjust to everything happening backward. But left-handers' advantages in life tend to stop right there.

Left-handed people get hassled by everything from common household tools to immune system problems. Let's face it. Left-handers live in a right-handed world. From a southpaw point of view, scissors cut the wrong way, corkscrews screw the wrong way, and using a power saw is a life-threatening experience. If that weren't enough, they've apparently got to deal with more auto-immune disease than the rest of the population.

"Left-handers get bad press. Especially from right-handers," says Alan Searleman, Ph.D., associate professor of psychology at St. Lawrence University, Canton, New York, and expert in the medical puzzles of left-handedness.

Left-handers' "bad press" goes way back. Even the scientific term for left-handedness – *sinistral* – comes from the same Latin root word as "sinister," Dr. Searleman points out. While the term for right-handedness – *dextral* – comes from the same Latin root as the word "dexterous."

"SINISTER" IMMUNE SYSTEMS

Dr. Searleman's studies of left-handedness confirm earlier findings that groups suffering from certain autoimmune diseases tend to have a larger proportion of left-handers than does the general population.

Left-handers are more likely to have an autoimmune disease than right-handers.

Approximately 10 percent of the general population is left-handed. But when Dr. Searleman questioned hundreds of people who have inflammatory bowel disease, he found that many more were left-handed than would be expected. In fact, more than 25 percent of the people with inflammatory bowel disease were left-handed. And among males, at least, Dr. Searleman found a left-handed link with juvenile-onset diabetes. Slightly more than 18 percent of men with that disease were left-handed.

Left-handers' immune system problems may start in the womb. According to this theory, an excess of the male sex hormone testosterone at the time of fetal development causes retarded growth in the left hemisphere of the brain, which accounts for the left-handedness and also suppresses the thymus, an important immune system organ.

An excess of male hormones may trigger both left-handedness and autoimmune disease.

"The theory is still controversial," says Dr. Searleman. But, he adds, the fact that left-handers with autoimmune disease are more likely to be males lends some credence to the idea.

SOUTHPAW DRUG REACTIONS

Nor are left-handers' medical differences limited to autoimmunity. It seems left-handed people may also be more sensitive to drugs that act on the central nervous system.

In studies that measured people's sensitivity to such drugs, brain electrical activity was greater in left-handers, according to Peter Irwin,

Left-handers may react more strongly than others to antidepressants, antihistamines, analgesics, and antianxiety drugs.

The dosage of prescription drugs should be tailored to each individual.

clinical research scientist at Sandoz Research Institute in East Hanover, New Jersey.

Irwin found that his left-handed study subjects reacted more strongly to sedating drugs that include antidepressants, antihistamines, analgesics, and antianxiety drugs.

"I found a very strong correlation between the degree of left-handedness and the magnitude of this reaction," says Irwin.

"These data do not yet have a clinical application," he says. "The only relevance this may have, if supported by further evidence, might be a greater awareness on the part of the physician when the patient is left-handed."

Doctors tend to tailor drug doses to individual patients in any case, says Irwin.

Are there any consolations, besides having an edge over your bowling partner, to being left-handed?

"Right-handers are like gingerbread men. If you've seen one you've seen them all," quips Dr. Searleman. "Neurologically speaking, left-handers are more interesting. There are a lot more of them with I.Q.'s above 140 than you would expect by chance."

29

LYME DISEASE: ARTHRITIS FROM TICKS

Lyme disease, a type of arthritis, appears to be spreading across the country like wildfire. But Lyme disease isn't new.

"Lyme disease does appear to be spreading," says medical epidemiologist Lee Harrison, M.D., of the Centers for Disease Control, "but it's difficult to tell if that's due to an actual spread or to increased reporting." There were about 1,400 cases reported in the United States in 1986, but that's "probably only a small fraction of the true number," Dr. Harrison says.

Although it's named after Lyme, Connecticut, where an outbreak occurred in 1975, the disease was known in Europe at the turn of the century. Caused by bacteria, Lyme is known for its ability to dwell in the body for several years and induce arthritis in its late stages. In most cases, it's completely curable with antibiotics.

Lyme disease was known in Europe at the turn of the century.

Lyme disease has been called the great imitator for its ability to mimic other diseases. "Many doctors aren't familiar with the symptoms," Dr. Harrison says, "which is why they don't report it as Lyme disease." In early stages, it's been misdiagnosed as meningitis, Bell's palsy, and sciatica.

Lyme has been called the great imitator for its ability to mimic other diseases.

According to immunologist Raymond Dattwyler, M.D., assistant professor of medicine at the State University of New York at Stony Brook, who is one of the nation's foremost Lyme researchers and clinicians, "It's become apparent that it's a much broader spectrum of disease than was originally thought."

A CLEVER LITTLE CONNIVER

Lyme disease is caused by a type of bacteria called a spirochete. In Lyme, the bacteria, *Borrelia burgdorferi,* is spread by the deer tick, a pinhead-size bloodsucker you can pick up while hiking and camping.

Borrelia is one of those microbes that is able to outwit the immune system, though it's not for lack of effort on the part of your immune system. Borrelia appears to have several ways of evading and neutralizing the immune system.

It's possible for Lyme to develop the personality of an autoimmune disease.

People with Lyme disease can have an imbalance between their helper T-cells and their suppressor T-cells within the affected joints. A State University of New York study showed higher numbers of helpers in the joint fluid of Lyme patients. Among the helpers' many duties is helping B-cells make antibodies. It's possible, Dr. Dattwyler says, that with so many helpers, antibody production in the joint fluid gets out of control, leading to the type of chronic inflammation typical of Lyme disease and rheumatoid arthritis. In other words, Dr. Dattwyler says, it's possible that Lyme can develop the personality of an autoimmune disease.

Further evidence of possible autoimmunity in Lyme came from a German research team. They showed that in the test tube, Borrelia can get T-cells to react against the body's own nervous system.

On the other hand, inadequate early treatment with antibiotics may also upset the antibody process, Dr. Dattwyler says.

The scenario goes like this: As they're supposed to do, microbe-eating macrophages show bits of their meal – called antigens – to a helper

T-cell, saying, "Look what I ate! Isn't it *disgusting?*" The T-cell heartily agrees, then starts reproducing itself, keeping the memory of that antigen. The T-cell tells a B-cell to get busy and clone itself and include that antigen memory in all the clones. The B-cell clone then goes back to the T-cell and proves it still remembers the microbe, and the T-cell says, "Okay, go ahead and start making antibodies to that miserable Lyme microbe."

But here's the catch: Dr. Dattwyler says that antibiotics may kill so many microbes that there aren't enough around for the immune system to recognize. The T-cell then won't tell the B-cell to make antibodies, and the B-cells don't grow up to be good little antibody makers. And the miserable microbe keeps on making you miserable.

Meanwhile, because the antibiotics didn't get all the bacteria, the conniving little germs may sneak their way into the central nervous system, where the immune system has very few troops and where antibody concentrations are lower. Here the bacteria can reproduce and begin causing the second-stage neurological symptoms.

Neurological symptoms develop in the second stage of the disease.

Interleukin-1 (IL-1) may have a central role in the development of Lyme disease, Dr. Dattwyler says. IL-1 is the messenger hormone macrophages send to T-cells. That hormone tells them, "Start cloning, we're under attack!" Borrelia does a really good job of getting macrophages to churn out IL-1, at least in the test tube.

Interleukin-1 may have a central role in the development of Lyme disease.

In turn, IL-1 stimulates the inflammation process that destroys cartilage and bones in an arthritic joint. "IL-1 also causes indirect destruction by revving up the immune system and creating a more intensive immune response," Dr. Dattwyler says. A hallmark of immune response is inflammation.

Natural killer (NK) cells are to certain bacteria what Tasmanian devils are to wombats. But unlike other bacteria that actually start NK cells on a killing rampage, Borrelia can severely inhibit an NK cell's murderous ability, Dr. Dattwyler says. But T-cells may be able to counteract Borrelia by releasing interleukin-2, a messenger which tells the killer T-cell, to take over the Kiss-of-Death Division of Immunity.

THE BAD, THE GOOD, AND THE ANTIBIOTICS

"The immune system is not necessarily capable of clearing the body of the organism," one doctor says.

All this evidence shows your immunity may not have what it takes to win the Lyme war. "As in syphilis, the immune system is not necessarily capable of clearing the body of the organism," Dr. Dattwyler says.

"We don't know why. These bacteria have evolved strategies to evade the immune system. Perhaps they can look like normal host proteins or normal cell surfaces. It's part of the typical repertoire of tricks that other microorganisms have evolved."

The lack of knowledge about Lyme plagues the development of therapies for it – a vaccine, for instance. How is the search for a vaccine coming? "Slowly," Dr. Dattwyler says. "There's nothing on the horizon yet. We don't really have very good funding."

Despite the problems, "the prognosis is definitely quite good," Dr. Dattwyler says. "It's actually very much like the prognosis for early syphilis. If you get treated promptly, you do very well. Treatment has a marked impact on abolishing the late-stage arthritis."

Dr. Dattwyler believes that the standard low-dose treatments of oral tetracycline or penicillin "are not acceptable. You need more and higher doses to wipe it out."

Lyme isn't deadly, he says. For the most part, it's more of a chronic, debilitating disease that can last several years. With antibiotics it is curable. The various inflammations of the brain and spinal cord and the inflammatory arthritis, "can make you miserable," he says, "but they're not lethal."

Early recognition and treatment are essential with Lyme disease, say Dr. Harrison and Dr. Dattwyler. Certain people are at risk for it, Dr. Dattwyler says. "It's a disease of healthy, active people who go places where they can get exposed to it."

Early recognition and treatment are essential.

Dr. Harrison realizes that hikers aren't going to wear long pants and long-sleeved shirts on a summer hike in 90-degree weather. "And I'm not recommending that people not go hiking in certain areas. But they should monitor themselves for ticks." He notes the deer tick is not your typical tick: It's only the size of a pinhead and may look like a speck of dirt.

Hikers need to watch for ticks, which cause Lyme disease, and know the early signs of the disease.

So it's helpful to know especially the early manifestations of the disease. Anywhere from three days to a month after you've been bitten by the tick, you may develop a small red pimple at the site, which expands over a few days to become a large rash. It can reach 6 inches in diameter, and as it grows it may begin to clear in the center and resemble a bull's-eye. This is when you should see a doctor and start getting antibiotics, but researchers say 20 to 40 percent either don't develop a rash or don't remember having one.

Other symptoms throughout the course of the disease, which can be several years, include fatigue, headache, stiff neck, morning stiffness, swollen lymph glands, and muscular pain.

Without adequate early treatment, the disease may progress into further stages. In its second stage, Lyme can cause central nervous system or cardiovascular problems like heart palpitations. These symptoms are like those of other diseases, so if you suspect Lyme because of your hike a few weeks or months ago, tell the doctor so diagnostic tests can focus on finding antibodies to it.

Arthritis can appear in the third stage, an average of a year after you contract the disease, and can last for several years. About 50 percent of patients do get chronic arthritis, which begins as intermittent joint pains. Once the arthritis is in full swing, the inflammation may begin to eat away at the joint. In some, the arthritis just goes away; others need antibiotics. Fortunately, once the disease is diagnosed, Dr. Dattwyler says, the prognosis is good.

30

NUTRITION: FEEDING THE TROOPS

Midnight strikes and the refrigerator beckons. It hums a seductive tune that promises late-night nibbles, and you waltz on over to see what's making that music. Light spills out onto the linoleum as you survey the grazing potential. Hmmm, a piece of chocolate cake, a six-pack of cola, some leftover pizza . . . What, no carrots? No crunchy bell pepper slices? No broccoli florets? How depressing!

Not depressing for *you*, who grabs at gastronomic pleasures with two-fisted gusto, but depressing for your immune system? Perhaps.

You know how you feel when you get depressed? You get the blahs and even though there's work to be done you could sum up your attitude toward duty with one word: *later*. And when you do get up the gumption to do what needs doing, you sort of half-heartedly take a stab at it.

It would be a sorry state of affairs if your immune system felt that way about fighting off invading viruses and stomping out tumor cells. ("Not now, man, I'm depressed.")

In a very real sense, that's what could happen if you never eat your veggies. You probably don't want to hear this. Your mother always nagged you to eat your vegetables. Now here you are, all grown up, and immunology researchers and doctors are telling you the same thing. There's no escape.

Your eating habits can depress your immune system.

207

GO FOR THE VEGGIES

A nutritious, well-balanced diet is absolutely vital.

A nutritious, well-balanced diet is absolutely vital to your immune system. And the single most important thing most people can do to improve their nutrition is to eat more vegetables, says Susanna Cunningham-Rundles, Ph.D., associate professor of immunology at Cornell Medical Center.

Most people really need to eat more vegetables.

"Most people's ideas of adequate vegetable quantities are probably a lot smaller than what really would be needed," says Dr. Cunningham-Rundles. "Clearly we know very little yet about specific recommendations for individual people – in terms of what might be needed to offset inborn problems in immune response. But it is important to recognize that diet should be taken seriously and not just left to chance or the spur of the moment. There's no question but what in the long run a great deal can be gained by diet."

The eat-and-run lifestyle that is so prevalent these days takes its toll on your whole body, creating stress, fatigue, and possible shortages of important nutrients. Is that any way to treat the cellular troops of your immune system? Would you expect an army to march on inadequate C rations? Would you ask soldiers to do battle on fast food lunches and TV dinners?

Almost any significant deficiency of any nutrient is likely to lower immunity.

"Almost any significant deficiency of any nutrient is likely to be immunosuppressive," says Ronald R. Watson, Ph.D., research professor from the University of Arizona's Department of Family and Community Medicine.

Of course, the key word here is "significant." Researchers know that your immune system is suppressed if you are so vitamin C deficient that you are approaching scurvy, or so lacking in vitamin A that you have night blindness, says Dr. Watson. But they still don't have a handle on that gray area where nutrient intakes are merely marginal. How deficient do you have to be before your immune system begins to feel the effects?

And just how much of which nutrients do you need in order to infuse your immune system with radiant health?

PIECES OF THE PUZZLE

Your immune system is not up to par? "Take two carrots and call me in the morning."

Dream on. Maybe *someday* in the not-too-distant future you will be able to visit a specialist who will prescribe a diet for your specific immune system needs. Someday. Right now, there is no one who can write such a prescription. The research isn't there.

Researchers are still working on individual pieces of the puzzle that will eventually come together to form the whole picture. Scattered around the country in separate laboratories, one research team is looking into zinc, while another examines the role of selenium. This researcher knows fats, that one can tell you all about vitamin B_6. They know a lot, and we'll summarize some of their findings for you shortly.

Meanwhile, you still want some general guidance on what to eat to keep your immune system humming at top efficiency.

At this point, the best advice is still to eat a well-balanced diet, says Dr. Cunningham-Rundles. And more specifically, it looks like the diet that experts recommend for fighting heart disease and preventing cancer may also be good for your immune system. That is, you want to go for a diet that is high in fiber, low in fat, and rich in whole grains, fruits, and vegetables.

The diet recommended by heart disease and cancer experts may be good for your immune system.

DIETERS BEWARE

One might think that in such a prosperous country, most folks would enjoy a more than adequate food intake to fuel the vital disease-preventing activities of their immune systems.

People on diets and the elderly may be starving their immune systems.

But it is precisely because so many people are struggling to cut calories that problems arise, says Dr. Watson. Even teenagers, whose healthy immune systems function with youthful vigor, can suppress their immune functioning if they don't eat enough of the right foods.

"If they're losing a lot of weight, if they're substantially below their weight, or if they're on a diet where they're taking less than 1,000 calories a day for some significant period of time, they may be protein-undernourished," says Dr. Watson. "That can be immunosuppressive.

"Also, all of these factors are more critical in the elderly. Their immune systems are damaged by age. They don't consume as much food, so they're not getting as many nutrients. Up to one-half of them are taking in less zinc than they should and probably eating less protein than they should. The elderly could certainly benefit from some sort of across-the-board vitamin and mineral supplement."

A multivitamin supplement is not a bad idea, provided it does not give people a false sense of security about their diets, says Dr. Cunningham-Rundles. Just don't use vitamin pills as a substitute for proper food choices, she warns.

OBESITY: A DIFFERENT DANGER

Obesity may suppress your immune system.

Dieting too strenuously can suppress your immune system. But that doesn't mean you can dive right into the next pie à la mode that crosses your path. It seems that obesity too may suppress your immune system.

There is no doubt that the immune systems of obese individuals are compromised, says Engikolai Krishnan, M.D., medical associate at the University of Kansas Medical Center. His own studies show that certain immune cells in obese people get ready for battle in much smaller numbers than do these cells in people of normal weight. Obese people also get more infections and are more likely to come down with some types of cancers. Whether it's the obesity itself, a related nutritional deficiency, or something else that causes the problems is not yet clear, says Dr. Krishnan.

Another study that looked at obese children and adolescents in a hospital setting found that 38 percent had impaired immune responses. Many of these children also proved to be deficient in either zinc or iron, two nutrients essential to the immune system.

Obesity in and of itself may not be the culprit when it comes to suppressing the immune response. Experts aren't yet sure. But if your bathroom scale screams when you step on it, you might want to ask yourself a little question as the loaded fork approaches your face for the umpteenth time: Do my macrophages and lymphocytes really need this pie?

NUTRIENTS YOUR IMMUNE SYSTEM NEEDS

Go for balance in your diet. Learn to love vegetables. And select a wide variety of foods. If you follow that basic advice, you'll probably meet your immune system's nutritional needs. Exactly what those needs are is a complex puzzle slowly being pieced together. Here's a simplified look at a few of the things your immune system has to have in order to carry out its vital functions.

Vitamin A. You've no doubt heard that vitamin A from carrots might help you avoid night blindness. That bit of nutritional wisdom has been floating around for decades. It's nice to know, but it's hardly the kind of stuff to make you elbow aside Bugs Bunny at the produce counter. What is currently coming out of research labs about the role that vitamin A plays in your immune system is, however. The carrot-munching rabbit had better stock in a good supply, because

Vitamin A, an anti-cancer vitamin, helps enhance immune functions.

it seems that orange, green, and yellow vegetables contain stuff that does a whole lot more than make you bright-eyed.

Scientists have known for years that vitamin A deficiency is linked to increased numbers of infections. More recent research shows that vitamin A helps enhance immune functions that have been suppressed by burns or surgical trauma. And the evidence is overwhelming that vitamin A is the number one anti-cancer vitamin. How could one nutrient do so much? What exactly does vitamin A do for your immune system?

While researchers don't yet have the whole answer to those questions, they do have lots of little answers. Vitamin A helps maintain the integrity of your skin and mucous membranes, both of which serve as your body's first-line barriers against invading microbes. In experimental animals, a diet deficient in vitamin A reduces the size of the spleen and thymus, both important immune system organs. Vitamin A is necessary for the maturation of some immune system cells and plays a role in stimulating these cells to repel invaders. Vitamin A also stimulates your immune system's production of certain antibodies. The list goes on. Researchers are especially interested in the cancer-fighting potential of this multi-faceted vitamin.

Beta-carotene seems to have almost no side effects.

"Our animal studies show that high vitamin A stimulates the immune system and reduces cancer," says the University of Arizona's Dr. Watson. "Whether this also occurs in people and whether there are any other side effects, it may be too early to say. But there is some suggestion that it might. Beta-carotene seems to be stimulating to the human immune system and seems to have almost no side effects."

Beta-carotene is a precursor of vitamin A that is found in carrots, broccoli, and most yellow and dark green leafy vegetables. Your body turns it into vitamin A. Preformed vitamin A, on the other hand, is found in liver, dairy products, and other animal foods. The U.S. Recommended Daily Allowance for vitamin A is 4,000 international units (IU) for women to 5,000 IU for men. Excessively high doses of vitamin A – 25,000 IU a day over a period of months – are toxic. But the only side effect one has to worry about from high doses of beta-carotene is changing color. According to Dr. Watson, if you take too much, your skin will turn yellow.

"Getting beta-carotene from fruits and vegetables would be the ideal choice, because you then get a lot of other benefits," says Dr. Watson. "There's nothing wrong with supplementing, but if you eat fruits and vegetables you get fiber, you get a low-fat diet, and you get a variety of other things that are beneficial to your body and your immune system.

Getting beta-carotene from fruits and vegetables would be ideal.

B vitamins. Remember those great old "health food" staples – wheat germ and blackstrap molasses? If these two foods don't tickle your fancy, how about liver and brown rice?

If you haven't guessed by now, we're talking about foods rich in vitamin B_6, possibly the most important B vitamin for your immune system's healthy functioning. That is to say, deficiencies in this particular nutrient seem to have a greater impact on your immune system than any other B deficiency.

Vitamin B_6 is possibly the most important B vitamin for your immune system.

Both human and animal studies at Oregon State University have shown that vitamin B_6 plays an important role in the immune system, says associate professor Nancy Kerkvliet, Ph.D. Laboratory animals deficient in vitamin B_6 don't produce as many antibodies. And the B_6-deficient animals make a poor showing in fighting off virus-induced tumors. Human immune systems also need this vital nutrient.

"Immune function has been shown to decline with age. Many older people are at risk of multiple vitamin deficiencies, but B_6 is one that they are particularly susceptible to," says Dr. Kerkvliet. "There might be more factors than

Elderly people are susceptible to vitamin B_6 deficiency.

poor intake. For some aged populations their B_6 intake is actually adequate. But they may not absorb it as well as younger people."

"Since vitamin B_6 deficiency in animals has been shown to result in impaired immunity, we asked the question: Could vitamin B_6 supplementation improve the immune response of elderly persons who were otherwise in good health? We found that the response could be improved."

Elderly people who took the B_6 supplements had a greater lymphocyte response to immune system challenges. The lymphocytes are white blood cells that attack invading bacteria and viruses.

Deficiencies of some of the other B vitamins are also associated with lower antibody production and poor lymphocyte response.

Vitamin C. There's a reason for that orange juice in the morning, and for the spinach nestled on your dinner plate. Actually, there are many reasons to enjoy fruits and vegetables, but getting enough vitamin C is surely one very good reason.

Just about every immunologic function works better in the presence of vitamin C.

"Just about any immunologic function that anybody's ever studied works better in the presence of vitamin C," says Jeffrey Delafuente, associate professor of pharmacy and medicine at the University of Florida. Delafuente's own studies too, have demonstrated that vitamin C enhances immune defenses.

Not only are the concentrations of vitamin C inside certain immune cells quite high, but the amount of vitamin C inside the cells actually decreases as cells do their infection-fighting work.

Your need for vitamin C may actually go up when you are sick.

You need adequate amounts of vitamin C even when you are healthy, but it looks as though your need for this vital nutrient may actually go up when you are sick. A Temple University study showed that invading bacteria secrete substances into the body that interfere with the absorption of vitamin C. These bacterial endotoxins increase a person's vitamin C requirements during illness, says Harish Padh, Ph.D., now research associate/ assistant professor at the University of Chicago Medical School.

So, if you feel that cold coming on, maybe you *should* reach for second helpings of your favorite vitamin C-rich fruits and vegetables. Go for that baked potato, a slice of ripe cantaloupe, a tall glass of freshly squeezed orange juice.

Vitamin D. Until recently, researchers were in the dark about the role that the sunshine vitamin plays in your immune system. Even now, there are just a few glimmers of light, but it stands to reason that a vitamin needed for strong bones might somehow have an impact on immune function. The bone marrow is, after all, the nursery for all the cells of your immune system.

Children with a vitamin D deficiency develop rickets, a condition characterized by thinning bones. They are also more susceptible to infection and have "depressed phagocytosis," according to one study. Phagocytes are the amoebalike immune cells that patrol your body on the lookout for anything that doesn't belong there. When they gobble up invading bacteria, that's phagocytosis. You don't want them sitting down on the job (assuming that amoebas can sit.)

Children with vitamin D deficiency have "depressed phagocytosis."

Drink your fortified milk for vitamin D and get a little sunshine every day. One note of caution. Elderly people who use sunscreens may not be getting enough vitamin D. Older people are prone to dietary vitamin D deficiency and frequently rely on sun exposure as their main source of this important nutrient. Yet even a single application of sunscreen can block the production of vitamin D. If you cover yourself with sunscreen when you face the sun, make sure your vitamin D needs are met elsewhere.

Vitamin E. Think you're getting enough vitamin E? If you're merely taking in the Recom-

The RDA for vitamin E may not be high enough for an aging immune system.

mended Dietary Allowance (RDA) for vitamin E, that might not be sufficient, says Jeffrey Blumberg, Ph.D., associate director of the U.S. Department of Agriculture's (USDA) Tufts Nutrition Center. Dr. Blumberg is studying the effects of vitamin E on the immune system. And what he has found so far has caused him to question whether the RDA for vitamin E is set high enough to maintain immune function as we age.

"Researchers noticed some time ago that vitamin E deficiency was associated with depressed immune responses. The work that I've done has shown that adequate, and even more interestingly, above normal levels of vitamin E seem to not only maintain, but boost immune function," says Dr. Blumberg.

"One thing that's been established repeatedly in both animals and humans is that immune function declines with age. And that decline seems to be associated with increased incidence of infectious diseases. When elderly people get sick, it takes them a lot longer to get better than younger individuals because their immune systems are not quite so vigorous.

High levels of vitamin E reverse the decline in immune function in laboratory animals.

"By giving old laboratory animals high levels of vitamin E in their diets, we found that we literally reversed the decline in immune function. We got an immunostimulation with vitamin E, and the reversal was so dramatic in many cases as to make the old animals indistinguishable from the young ones."

Vitamin E may regulate the immune system's on/off switch.

It is possible that vitamin E affects the immune system by putting the dampers on the body's production of a hormonelike compound known as prostaglandin 2 (PGE_2). PGE_2 is one of the compounds that regulates immune function. It serves as a type of off switch for the immune system, says Dr. Blumberg.

"When we gave vitamin E, we found that it depressed the production of PGE_2. It seems that vitamin E inhibits the inhibitor. When you turn an off switch off, the response is on," he says.

In elderly animals, getting enough vitamin E seems to keep the aging immune system in its switched-on condition. Dr. Blumberg is now working on clinical studies with elderly human volunteers to see whether the same will hold true for them. If it does, he says, it may lead eventually to revamping the RDA for vitamin E.

Meanwhile, how much vitamin E should we try to get? Dr. Blumberg gets his vitamin E from a multivitamin supplement that meets or exceeds the current RDA for vitamin E. The current RDA is 10 to 20 IU. Dr. Blumberg does not recommend taking high doses of vitamin E. Indeed, some studies have shown that very high levels seem to suppress immune function. The best food sources for vitamin E are vegetable oils.

Calcium. Calcium plays a role in activating complement. Complement is a series of proteins that work with antibodies to explode invading bacteria. (And you thought calcium was just for building strong bones!) Good food sources of this mineral include low-fat milk, low-fat yogurt, and other dairy products.

Calcium plays a role in activating complement.

Copper. Besides making pretty teapots and conducting electricity to your household appliances, copper performs an essential but little understood function in your immune system. Researchers don't know exactly how copper does its stuff, but they do know what happens if you don't get enough of it, says Timothy R. Kramer, Ph.D., research immunologist for the USDA's Human Nutrition Research Center.

Copper performs an essential function in your immune system.

"Without copper, your T-lymphocytes are not working at optimum, which means you have an increased chance of infection. It also means that your protection against tumor development is weakened," says Dr. Kramer.

There are also a few studies indicating that the production of interleukin-2 is decreased if you don't get enough copper. Interleukin-2 is an important chemical messenger for your immune system.

Getting enough copper is just one more reason to eat your beans, because legumes are a rich source of this essential nutrient.

Iron. America's number one nutritional deficiency problem may be iron depletion. You've no doubt heard that lack of iron causes that dragged-out, no-energy feeling. Without iron, your immune system also loses its pep.

Lack of iron interferes with your neutrophils and T-cells.

If your neutrophils don't get enough iron, they can still manage to do their job of gobbling up invading bacteria. The problem is, once they eat them, they can't digest them as well.

Without sufficient iron, there are also fewer circulating T-cells, the white blood cells that patrol your body on the lookout for invading viruses. And the T-cells that *are* out there can't perform as well as they should if you are iron-deficient.

Iron-deficient laboratory animals were found to have smaller spleens. The spleen is an important organ used as a sort of garrison for the warrior cells of the immune system. And the animals' natural killer (NK) cells weren't as energetic. NK cells eradicate some kinds of cancer cells.

The many ways that iron supports the activities of your immune system may make you wonder how to get the iron out of your frying pan and into your food. Actually, just using an iron skillet puts some additional iron into your food. Other good sources of iron include liver, spinach, beef, sunflower seeds, and beans.

Magnesium is needed for lymphocyte growth.

Magnesium. Magnesium deficiency depresses the body's levels of most immunoglobulins, antibodies important in disease prevention. The mineral is also needed for lymphocyte growth. Food sources include nuts and whole grains.

Selenium also is vital.

Selenium. Selenium is found nestled in the table of chemical elements between arsenic and bromine. That's an odd place to find a cancer-fighting substance. Ask a selenium researcher how this micronutrient fights cancer and the answer is something along the lines of "it stimulates the immune system." The role of selenium in immune functioning is not yet clear, but there are some hints.

Selenium and vitamin E seem to work hand in hand. Studies show that if both are deficient or absent from the diet of chicks, the birds' ability to produce antibodies is reduced.

Infection-fighting T-cells also seem to need an adequate supply of selenium in order to be activated.

The RDA for selenium is 50 to 200 micrograms per day. Too much is toxic. Foods rich in selenium include whole wheat bread, liver, rice, and tuna.

Zinc. Want to put more power in your immune system's punch? Then take an oyster to dinner. Take several oysters. All of this talk of seafood should make you think zinc. And as you get older, you should think zinc even more because your immune system's need for this essential nutritional element may be even more critical as you age.

It seems that everything in your immune system needs zinc.

As research piles up on the zinc connection, it begins to look like there's nothing in your immune system that *doesn't* need zinc.

"Zinc is essential for the biological activity of thymic hormone," says Dr. Cunningham-Rundles. "The thymus is a gland which is quite large in children, but diminishes and atrophies as we grow older. People over the age of 20 begin to show a diminishing size of the thymus gland. We know that the thymus has an important role in the maturation of T-cells, which are a very important component in the immune system."

"It seems that the role of zinc in later life may be even more important than it is in children, when the gland is larger. Zinc makes the thymic hormone itself more biologically active. And in

A zinc supplement might be a good idea for the elderly.

the absence of normal amounts of zinc, thymic hormone is not as active. So zinc is necessary for the maturation and complete development of T-cells. There have been studies suggesting that in the aging population, the addition of zinc supplements has been valuable in improving immune response."

Everything from the thymus to the NK cells requires zinc.

Your thymus thrives on zinc. Your virus-fighting T-cells need zinc to do their stuff. Your neutrophils, the cells that are your immune system's first line of defense, apparently need their zinc. Your NK cells, the ones that zap cancer cells, may also need their zinc. Studies show that NK cells in zinc-deficient animals are not as active as they should be.

With all these different types of cells and enzymes making their demands for zinc, you want to make sure there is enough to go around. You wouldn't want any of the cellular troops to come up short. So, how much is enough?

The RDA for zinc is 15 milligrams a day, and up to six times that amount is considered safe. Although some studies have shown that excessive amounts of zinc can suppress some immune system functions, the amounts were far beyond what one would take in normal supplementation, says Dr. Cunningham-Rundles. She recommends a 50 milligram-a-day zinc supplement, especially for the elderly.

31

PARASITES:
THE BIGGEST OF THE BAD GUYS

A rugged camper sips water in the high Colorado Rockies. A Brooklyn housewife samples the gefilte fish she's preparing. A barefoot child runs across a backyard in the rural South. A young stockbroker savors a morsel of sushi. And Grandma proudly sets her Christmas sausage (it's just a trifle pink) on the family table.

It all seems innocent enough. But all of these people are engaging in behavior that might bring them in contact with a parasitic infestation.

Bacteria and viruses are not the only creatures that move right into the human body and make themselves at home. There are other things that your immune system has to guard against – parasites that range in size from the tiny protozoa that squeeze into red blood cells and cause malaria to the tapeworm that enters the body via uncooked fish and can grow up to (*ugh!*) 30 feet in length.

It's not a pretty subject. But it's so very easy to avoid contact with these unsavory creatures that a brief consideration of the matter is appropriate.

AMERICA,
THE (ALMOST) PARASITE-FREE

Actually, the chances of contracting a serious parasitic infection in North America are

221

relatively slim. Compared to the rest of the world, America is blessed with a dearth of predatory parasites according to Richard Davidson, M.D., associate professor at the University of Florida College of Medicine.

"Parasitic infections worldwide cause more deaths each year than cancer, stroke, and heart disease put together," says Dr. Davidson.

But not here.

People with healthy immune systems usually don't have to worry.

While third world countries contend with parasitic scourges like schistosomiasis (acquired from snails in wet places like rice paddies) and malaria, most Americans share their space with only a few relatively benign parasites. And our immune systems are so good at dispatching these parasites that we *do* encounter on a regular basis, that for all intents and purposes the nasty creatures might as well not exist.

If you doubt that, just consider the threats facing people with compromised immune systems, says Stewart Duncan, Ph.D., professor of biology and public health at Boston University. People with AIDS often die of pneumocystic pneumonia, a form of the lung disease caused by parasites. They are also sometimes ravaged by toxoplasmosis, a normally harmless parasitic infection carried by domestic cats.

"The parasites are just waiting there, lurking," says Dr. Duncan. People with healthy immune systems don't usually have to worry about them, but immunocompromised people are sitting ducks.

For the North American with a normally functioning immune system, however, a few parasitic threats do exist – but further from the beaten track.

Fortunately, taking a few precautions erects a protective barrier. Here's what you can do.

A CAMPER'S STORY

Camper, beware.

That clear, cold water that looks so very appealing running in a high mountain stream is not necessarily as pure as you might think. It's so easy to be lulled into a false sense of security. The mountains are high. The source of the water is spring snow run-off. What possible pollution source could there be?

What we're worried about at that crystal stream is not man-made pollution but beaver-made parasites. Wherever you have beaver (or even other campers who are careless about where they defecate), you can have giardia.

Giardia lamblia are tiny one-celled animals – protozoa – that can cause very big diarrhea problems and stomachaches so bad you'll think you're not going to make it.

No, you don't take a sip of water and keel over. There is a latency period of approximately one week before you notice the symptoms. By the time the giardia goes to work, the camping trip is only a memory.

If you're lucky, the ingested giardia will cause only mild diarrhea. But a hefty dose causes "explosive" diarrhea that goes on and on. It is even possible to get a chronic giardia disease that lasts for months or years.

The cure for giardia is prescription drugs, says Dr. Davidson. To get rid of it, you'll have to visit your physician.

It's so much easier not to get it in the first place.

Giardia precaution number one: Never, ever, *ever* drink water from a stream without first boiling it.

Boiling kills giardia. Interestingly enough, chlorination does not. Some cities are plagued

You can catch giardia from a clear mountain stream.

Symptoms range from mild diarrhea to a chronic disease that lasts for months.

with giardia in the municipal water supply. Leningrad in the Soviet Union has a major giardia problem, for example. But it isn't necessary to travel that far to encounter the little beasts, says Dr. Davidson. Parts of Pennsylvania suffered a major outbreak a few years ago.

Giardia precaution number two: When traveling in foreign countries, unless you are absolutely sure of the water supply, don't drink the water. Use bottled water or some other bottled beverage. If your own city sometimes experiences giardia problems, switch to bottled water.

If you have doubts about the water, boil it.

A PIG STORY

This little piggy went to market. But he wasn't alone. Hitching a ride inside every pork chop and bacon slab in his tender little body were a number of worms.

Remember when your mother warned you about pork? "Cook pork until the pink goes away," she cautioned.

Mom was right. With a vengeance.

Pigs raised in the United States are sometimes infected with *Trichinella spiralis*.

Pigs raised in the United States are sometimes infected with *Trichinella spiralis,* which causes trichinosis, according to William Campbell, Ph.D., senior director of basic parasitology at Merck Institute for Therapeutic Research. Not all pigs are infected, not by any means, but the problem is serious enough that many European and Asian countries will not import American pork.

"We have never effectively tested pork for the protection of the American consumer. The old test methods were considered unsuitable, but new methods are being developed," says Dr. Campbell.

There are far fewer cases of trichinosis than there used to be.

Because of education about the dangers of undercooked pork, there are far fewer cases of trichinosis than there used to be. At the end of World War II, there were 300 to 400 cases a year reported in the United States, but in the 1980s there were fewer than 100 cases reported annually. These are the more severe, clinical cases, Dr. Campbell emphasizes. There are many more cases of trichinosis that go unreported because they are mild.

Trichinosis is caused by ingesting trichinella larvae, which grow up in the intestines. Their offspring leave the intestines and enter the muscles. A few worms may go unnoticed, but a large number can be extremely painful and even prove fatal.

The first phase of trichinosis consists of intestinal upset and diarrhea. The infection progresses from there to fever and excruciating muscle pain.

Again, the best way to deal with trichinosis is to not get it in the first place.

Prevention is the best way to deal with trichinosis.

"It's so *easy* to protect oneself," says Dr. Campbell. "Modern home freezers offer tremendous protection. Freezing kills trichinella, and so does cooking. If the pork is cooked until it's white and not pink, it's okay."

Homemade sausages from the farm are of particular concern. If you do sample these delicacies, make sure they are well cooked, done through and through without even a suggestion of pink.

One final note. Pigs are not the only animals that harbor trichinella. Some wild game, especially bear meat, is notorious. The same rules apply here – if you're going to eat it, make sure it's cooked until it's well done.

A FISH STORY

Raw and undercooked fish can also harbor parasites that cause infection. Although the problem is not severe in North American waters, it

It is possible to get parasites from raw and undercooked fish.

does exist, says Terry Dick, Ph.D., professor of zoology at the University of Manitoba.

At the turn of the century, it was not uncommon for women to ingest fish tapeworms while preparing gefilte fish, says Dr. Dick. They sampled the raw fish while they were making the delicacy, before it was fully pickled.

Cold smoked salmon and other raw fish can also harbor parasites. Does that mean you should stay away from sushi bars?

"If restaurants use good quality control in their selection of fish, it shouldn't be a problem," says Dr. Dick.

Both freezing and cooking kill fish parasites. When in doubt, cook it.

A CAT STORY

Almost anyone who owns a pet cat and tends kitty's litter box comes in contact with yet another protozoan – the microscopic creature that causes toxoplasmosis.

In general, toxoplasmosis is not ordinarily an important concern for adults. But there are important exceptions: Pregnant women and those whose immune systems are suppressed.

Toxoplasmosis is dangerous to pregnant women and people whose immune systems are suppressed.

"Most people have a good, strong, natural resistance to toxoplasmosis. It is estimated that 25 to 50 percent of the people in the United States have been exposed to it. Most don't show any symptoms," says Boston University's Dr. Duncan.

The real danger with toxoplasmosis is to pregnant women. If the parasite infects a woman while she is pregnant, the infection can kill her unborn child or cause blindness and other birth defects.

"Pregnant women should avoid cats as much as possible," advises Dr. Duncan.

If there is a pet cat in the household, a pregnant woman should not change the litter box, says Dr. Davidson. Let someone else take on that chore.

A CHILDREN'S STORY

We can't leave the subject of parasites without mentioning children and the assorted roundworms they can encounter – especially hookworms and pinworms.

Children come in contact with a number of parasites.

Children in the rural South still have to be checked for hookworm, which enters the body through the feet. And there is no part of the country that's free of pinworms. These little wigglies get passed from child to child in daycare centers and wherever else large numbers of toddlers come together. Apart from isolating your child at home, there is no way to prevent possible exposure.

Fortunately, pinworms are not dangerous, and the cure comes in the form of one little pill. If you notice that your child is suffering from anal itching, mention it to your pediatrician.

32

PESTICIDES:
THEIR EFFECT ON IMMUNITY

Homicide: the killing of a person.
Fratricide: the killing of one's brother.
Matricide: the killing of one's mother.
Pesticide: an agent that kills bugs.

Pesticides kill.

The common thread in this litany is the word *kill.* Pesticides kill. Most of us either don't realize – or just plain forget – that these products are agents of death.

And it's easy to forget. Pesticides are so commonplace and seem so normal. They line up like bright soldiers on the supermarket shelf. They stand among the honest rakes, hoes, and shovels at the garden center. They're packaged prettily and displayed beside the squeakie toys at the pet store. In our desire for a velvet, grub-free lawn, an American Beauty rose bush that can fend off an attacking squadron of Japanese beetles, a peach that looks like a Holbein painting, a house free of roaches and flies, and a dog without fleas, we sometimes simply forget that we are dealing with a killing product.

THE TRADE-OFF

And so we spray, dust, fog, and collar. There are no roaches skittering down the wall behind the stove in *our* house. The gloxinia is aphid-free, and there are no cucumber beetles among

228

our garden vines. But what price do we pay for our pest-free environment?

In some cases we have traded bugs on the vine for poison in our water, our food, and our air. And while you can see a Colorado potato beetle or a fat, ugly dog tick, you can't see the alar on the apples you eat. Or the chlordane in the air you breathe. It is possible that, in our quest for bug-free perfection, we may have traded in some of our body's resistance to disease. And just how much have we given away? Well, if you ask a doctor who practices environmental medicine (also called clinical ecology), he might say our immunity's cruisin' for a bruisin'.

We may have traded some of our body's resistance to disease in exchange for a bug-free society.

Immune systems were meant to handle viruses, bacteria, fungi, parasites, particles, and a lot of other onslaughts. Pesticides, however, were meant to overwhelm the defense systems of insects and other living things. Since World War II, 60,000 new chemicals – including pesticides – have flooded into the environment. Combine those with the millions of little enemies we evolved with and it's apparent we have something new to think about.

THE EVIDENCE IS THERE

The litany of pesticide-caused immune problems ranges from allergy to loss of disease resistance. All of these involve the white blood cells, the standing army of immunity. Allergies, especially skin inflammations (dermatitis), are the most common visible sign that pesticides are challenging your immune system. These reactions are most often found in farm and pesticide industry workers. But even if you just use pesticides on your garden or pet or roaches, the immune problems suffered by these workers should sound the alarm loud and clear.

Pesticides zap your immune system.

San Francisco immunologist Alan Levin, M.D., says people poisoned by pesticides commonly have an abnormal ratio of the helper T-cells to the suppressor T-cells. This abnormality negatively affects the immune system's efficiency.

For ethical reasons, most pesticide toxicity studies are performed on animals. Humans are studied only when they have already been exposed on the job, and it's hard to conduct valid studies this way. The lack of human studies, and the validity of applying the results of animal studies to humans, is at the core of the dispute between clinical ecologists and establishment medicine.

ALARMING ANIMAL STUDIES

But the immune systems of animals – from mouse to man – are similar in composition, says Gary Rosenthal, Ph.D., senior research scientist with the National Institute of Environmental Health Sciences. All have killer cells, B-cells, T-cells, and antibodies. (The way in which these cells respond when exposed to chemicals may be different.)

The similar composition of human and animal immune systems makes the results of the nonhuman animal studies cautionary, if not alarming.

Some pesticides seem to drain the very marrow from your bones.

- When animals are exposed to the pesticide carbofurans, their white blood cell counts drop along with bone marrow cell counts. Bone marrow, a primary organ of the immune system, makes white blood cells.
- Ethyl carbamate also damages bone marrow, keeps killer cells from efficiently killing tumor cells, bacteria, and other invaders, and cuts down on the numbers of antibody-producing B-cells.

- Carbaryl also depletes B-cell numbers, and in the test tube allows viruses to infect human lung cells.
- Methyl parathion depresses immunity and allows salmonella to become deadlier than it usually is, while dieldrin does the same for the hepatitis virus. Dieldrin also makes invader-eating macrophages less effective.
- The termite poison chlordane causes immune suppression for life in animals exposed to it while still in the womb.
- Dioxin, a contaminant of pentachlorophenol (PCP), is a highly potent immune suppressant and causes cancer of the immune system.

HOW ABOUT PEOPLE?

John Jones, a 55-year-old California farmer, had used pesticides throughout his career, with not the greatest caution. But one day in 1985 he siphoned his last mouthful of the insecticide Aldicarb. Days later his skin broke out in rashes, and over the next few weeks he developed an ominous mixture of immune and nervous system ailments. He is now "totally disabled," according to his doctor, Alan Levin. Farmer Jones (not his real name) has what Dr. Levin calls CAIDS – chemically acquired immune deficiency syndrome.

While the white blood cell count of a healthy person should be around 7,000, a person suffering from CAIDS "rarely has a white count over 5,500," he says. A healthy person should have 1.8 to 2 helper T-cells for each suppressor T-cell, but the CAIDS patient's ratio is usually below 1.4, which shows his immune system isn't turning on as well as it should and is turning off *too* well.

Contact with pesticides can lead to CAIDS—chemically acquired immune deficiency syndrome.

Some people feel like they have the flu, but they don't.

Some people, like farmer Jones, who have been exposed frequently to pesticides at low levels over long periods of time, develop "a gradual intolerance to environmental chemicals of all types," Dr. Levin says. "They feel like they have the flu all the time. Doctors find great similarity between their symptoms and those of people with acute infectious hepatitis." They become depressed and anxious and have abnormal blood counts and memory lapses, nausea, confusion, headaches – all of which suggests illness caused by weakened immunity.

Few of us, however, siphon pesticides or handle them as frequently as a farmer does. What is the danger for the weekend gardener or the bugophobic housekeeper?

For starters, a University of Southern California statistical study found that when parents used pesticides in the home or garden, they increased their children's risk of developing leukemia. Symptoms of leukemia include fever (an immune reaction), susceptibility to infections (a sign of depressed immunity), and enlargement of the lymph nodes and spleen (essential components of the immune system).

Your immune system has substantial reserves.

While studies of humans exposed to pesticides may show some effect on the immune system, Dr. Rosenthal says, "there's not enough evidence to say that a 3 or 4 percent change is enough to have an impact. The immune system has substantial reserve capacity. It can be suppressed considerably and still be able to eradicate a tumor."

There have been far too few "properly conducted clinical trials" to be able to say the weekend gardener or the household cockroach hunter is endangering his or her immunity, say some medical experts.

Maybe so, but taking some precautions when using pesticides – if you use pesticides – only makes common sense.

COMMONSENSE PEST CONTROL

Many "natural" techniques work effectively to control pests – flyswatters, ant traps, Japanese beetle bags, and sprays of soapy water. But if you're determined to use pesticides, use them with the thought that they are chemicals designed to kill. "We just need to use them in a less cavalier fashion," says Dr. Levin. "Prevention is the most important aspect. The solution is common sense."

The solution is common sense.

If you use pesticides, common sense means:

- Following directions. One teaspoon per gallon mcans 1 teaspoon per gallon. Two teaspoons isn't better, it's worse.
- Wearing gloves and a mask or respirator.
- Using pesticides indoors means "ventilate, ventilate, ventilate" says Dr. Levin.
- Disposing of the leftover pesticides, and their containers, properly.
- Helping your immune system to do its job by providing adequate nutrition, sleep, exercise, and relaxation.
- Taking care in using pesticides around the sick, the elderly, the pregnant, and the immune deficient.

33

PNEUMONIA: IT'S MEANER THAN YOU THINK

A cold by any other name can lay you low.

Chuck looked out the window of his hospital room and wondered if the day was as warm as it looked. He had gone into the hospital at the beginning of March when the wind still clawed at his parka and sent chills rippling across every inch of his 60-year-old body.

Now it was the beginning of April. And although the trees had not yet begun to bloom around the Pennsylvania hillside against which the hospital nestled, the sun was beginning to take its time crossing the sky, tulips and hyacinths were poking sturdy green shoots out of their winter mulch, and bright yellow crocuses were already dancing across the hospital's lawn.

It certainly looked warmer, Chuck thought. It might even be warm enough to plant the lettuce in the cold frame. He'd ask Jane – a paroxysm of coughing interrupted his thoughts – he'd ask Jane if maybe he should do it next week. Surely he'd be out of the hospital by then. If he could just shake this cold.

But Chuck never lived to plant his lettuce. He died two days after the cherry tree bloomed outside his window, three days after the pneumonia that had inflamed his lungs suddenly seemed to outmaneuver his immune system.

WHO IS AT RISK?

Pneumonia is an inflammation of the lungs that can be triggered by any one of a half-dozen

234

different viruses and bacteria that live around us every day. "And if you inhale a big enough dose, your body's natural protective responses can't eliminate them," says Kenneth L. Brigham, M.D., the Joe and Morris Werthan Professor of Investigative Medicine at Vanderbilt University School of Medicine's Center for Lung Research.

"That's why people who are otherwise ill" – people like Chuck – "are more susceptible," says Dr. Brigham. "Their host defenses are not as vigorous as normal. That's also why people with AIDS or flu or people who are being treated with chemotherapeutic agents for cancer die of pneumonia. Their natural defenses are suppressed.

People die of pneumonia when their immune systems are overwhelmed.

"Older people also have a less aggressive immune system than younger people," he adds. "So just age itself predisposes you to more infections. And any severe stress on the body, like a broken bone, would also reduce the body's ability to defend against infection."

Severe stress reduces the body's ability to defend itself.

A BACTERIA COOKOUT

How does your body normally defend itself from the viruses and bacteria that trigger pneumonia? "You have mucus in the upper airway that is balanced on top of cilia [hairs] that propel the mucus up the airway all the time," explains Dr. Brigham. "Things get stuck in this mucus and then they get transported out. They never get to the lower airways."

On the rare occasion when they do, says Dr. Brigham, "Your number one line of defense is a group of cells found in the lower airways called the alveolar macrophages.

Macrophages and neutrophils go after the microbes that cause pneumonia.

"Those cells, which actually live in air spaces within your lungs, engulf the bacteria. Inside the macrophage, enzymes kill the bacteria.

"If the macrophage can't get rid of the invader, it secretes some stuff that attracts the neutrophils, another type of [eater cell] from where it circulates in the blood. Then the neutrophils engulf the bacteria and fry them."

Fry them? What is this – a cookout? Dr. Brigham laughs. "Almost. The principal mechanism that a neutrophil uses to kill bacteria is the generation of oxidants, which are a highly reactive species of oxygen molecule. So since oxidation is 'fire,' if you use your imagination a little bit, you can say the netrophils 'fry' the bacteria." They burn it up with oxygen.

"In fact, that process – the neutrophils coming in – is called inflammation. So any time you have pneumonia," he adds, "you have a bunch of neutrophils in your lungs."

WHEN YOUR IMMUNE SYSTEM MAKES A MISTAKE

"Confused" neutrophils can cause pneumonia.

"But even neutrophils can make mistakes," says Dr. Brigham. And when they do, that can cause pneumonia, too. "One theory is that the neutrophils that are circulating in the blood get turned on. Instead of being aimed at a given site, they attack the entire lung. Then they generate these oxidants as though they were trying to kill bacteria – even without bacteria being there – and injure the cells that line the blood vessels.

"But my theory is that such an injury doesn't happen with *normal* endothelial cells – the cells that line the blood vessels – unless they're already injured. That first injury sends a message to the circulating neutrophils that the endothelial cells are 'not-self' – not a part of you. That's what causes the blood vessels in your lungs to be attacked.

"Then the neutrophil, which operates on a hair trigger, blows them up."

But what causes the initial injury? "What I think happens is that the endothelial cells are injured by an endotoxin – a kind of poison that's generated by any bacteria that may be floating around in your bloodstream. Then the neutrophils charge in to save the day and, like misguided commandos, blow up your lungs instead," explains Dr. Brigham.

PREVENTION AND PENICILLIN

Once you've got pneumonia, the treatment depends on the kind you've got, says Dr. Brigham. "Pneumococcal pneumonia, for example, is highly sensitive to prompt treatment with penicillin."

But penicillin won't save everybody. "Some organisms that cause pneumonia are highly resistant to a variety of antibiotics," says Dr. Brigham. "Pneumonias acquired in the hospital also tend to involve highly resistant organisms because they've been exposed to a variety of antibiotics in the hospital environment. They've built up a resistance." And viral pneumonias don't respond to antibiotics at all.

That's why prevention is of such paramount importance, Dr. Brigham emphasizes. Older people and people who have underlying respiratory problems should get both the pneumococcus vaccine and a flu shot. Each will protect them from getting at least one particular cause of pneumonia. Avoiding rooms full of cigarette smoke, which suppresses your lungs' immune defenses, as well as avoiding people who are ill, will help prevent the rest.

Had he known that, Chuck might be planting his lettuce.

Penicillin won't save everybody.

34

POLLUTION: LONG-TERM, LOW-LEVEL DANGER

What happens when man-made chemicals mix with the ones inside your body?

Each day, our immune systems are exposed to 40,000 chemicals in the workplace alone. Only 8,500 of them have been tested for their effect on health. And no one has discovered much about what they do when they *combine* with each other inside the body. Or what happens when they mix into the body's own formidable chemical factory.

"The immune system is resilient," says Linda D. Caren, Ph.D., associate professor of biology at California State University in Northridge. "Even transplant patients who take enormous doses of immunosuppressants can survive. But the immune system is also very complicated. You disturb one little part of it and who knows what checks and balances are brought into play?" That's why immunologists aren't sure about the *long-term* effects of living in a polluted environment.

Take air pollution, for example. "There's evidence that there's a higher incidence of some respiratory disorders in certain localities where there's a lot of smog," Dr. Caren says. "But you can't really say there is a direct cause-and-effect link between, say, the sulfur dioxide in smog and these disorders."

The science that studies these medical statistics is called epidemiology. It focuses on a population, in this case tracing their past exposure to a pollutant and trying to determine whether that group has an increased risk of

238

illness. Such studies are not definitive, but they are helpful.

"These studies can raise a red flag," says Dr. Caren. "On some bad days in Los Angeles, people's exposure to pollutants in smog does approach the levels in lab studies in which animals have been given cancer. People should especially look at their chemical exposure from occupations and hobbies. Chemists, for instance, have higher rates of some kinds of cancer. Be aware of the risks. It's prudent to limit your exposure."

Chemists are more likely to have some types of cancer.

POLLUTANTS TO WATCH FOR

Exposure to what? Several pollutants have been linked to an effect on the immunity of laboratory animals or humans.

Certain *metals* have been shown to weaken the immune system of lab animals by suppressing their antibody production. Lead, cadmium, mercury, cobalt, and arsenic all increased their susceptiblity to infection. Cadmium, for example, brought about immunosuppression, even in doses that didn't cause any signs of cadmium poisoning. Where might people encounter these heavy metals? Almost anywhere. Lead is in the air; cadmium is found in drinking water, many foods, cigarette smoke, and various industrial products; cobalt sulfate is often added to beer to stabilize foam; arsenic is found in pesticides, feed additives, and detergents.

Polychlorinated biphenyls (PCBs) are known to suppress the immune system. In laboratory animals, PCBs have atrophied the thymus cortex (home of the T-cells), reduced the number of sites in the spleen and lymph nodes where immune cells are stored, caused a drop in antibody production, cut the number of lymphocytes in the blood, and increased the death rate from infectious disease. PCBs can punch out your immune system without causing any signs

PCBs can punch out your immune system.

of PCB poisoning. PCBs are used in insulators, lubricants, paints, varnishes, and waxes. Like metals, they accumulate in the body.

Sulfuric acid, a component of urban air pollution, made it harder for test animals to rid their lungs of streptococcus bacteria. Another study showed higher rates of pneumonia in lab animals infected with the flu virus and then exposed to sulfuric acid aerosol.

Carbon monoxide can increase the numbers of neutrophils in the spleen, lungs, and lymph nodes of test animals, according to one Swedish study. The same study showed an increase in the number of lung macrophages. These phagocytes eat foreign particles for breakfast and as a by-product cause inflammation. So it's good that immune cells absorb carbon monoxide molecules but bad that inflammation can be the burp that follows the meal.

Nitrogen dioxide, a pollutant of natural gas, reduces the numbers of B-cells (which produce antibodies), but doesn't seem to suppress the immune response, according to investigators at Texas Tech Health Sciences Center. Other studies, however, found greater susceptibility to bacterial and viral infections.

The ozone in California smog may zap the macrophages that defend your lungs from invaders.

Ozone may slow down the proliferation of T-cells, according to the Environmental Protection Agency (EPA), which studied a small group of people who had been exposed to this gas. The study described the T-cells as "exquisitely sensitive" to ozone. The ozone level used in the study is often found on high-smog days in southern California. Probably the major pollutant of urban air, ozone is thought to cause cell damage through oxidation and the resulting free radicals. The EPA study said ozone may interfere with T-cells by oxidizing their cell wall surfaces. Ozone also seems to decrease numbers of lung macrophages and their ability to eat invaders.

"All in all," Dr. Caren says, "there's substantial evidence that gaseous pollutants produced by transportation, fuel combustion, industrial processes, or cigarette smoking could impair the immune response and may decrease resistance to infectious disease."

THE MOST DANGEROUS JOBS

Some jobs involve a greater potential exposure to pollutants than others. The National Institute for Occupational Safety and Health has extensively studied pollutant exposure on the job. Following is a sampling of occupations and workplaces where you may have contact with a large number of chemicals. The numbers of dangerous chemicals for each job are noted. Just keep in mind that the chemicals in one job may be fewer in number but more dangerous than in another.

- Hospitals: 658
- Janitors: 627
- Pharmaceutical preparation: 360
- Registered nurses: 300
- Business services (like photocopying): 282
- Automobile mechanics: 264
- Painters, construction workers, and maintenance people: 227
- Nursing aides, orderlies, attendants: 153
- Hairdressers and cosmetologists: 105
- Gasoline service stations: 96

PREVENTIVE ACTION

Exposure to a pollutant is an "insult" to the body. When the number of insults accumulates to a critical level, the immune system staggers under the burden. Obviously, the wisest action is to avoid these exposures in every practical way that you can: stay indoors during smog alerts, avoid cigarette and other smoke, use chemicals only in well-ventilated areas, and wear protective gloves when handling chemicals.

Stay inside during a smog alert, avoid cigarette smoke, and use chemicals only in well-ventilated areas.

35

RADIATION:
SUNSHINE THAT HURTS

The construction workers breaking up the roadway were masters of the universe. Stripped to the waist, they pulverized cement, crumbled stone, and melted macadam with the sheer force of hands, drills, hammers, and heat. Nothing could withstand their assault.

But their seeming invincibility didn't mean the workers were invulnerable. Far from it. Because while they were attacking the earth, the sun was attacking them.

Ultraviolet rays from the sun can trigger skin cancer.

Who was doing the most harm? It's a toss-up. Construction workers may be able to move the earth, but ultraviolet waves radiating from the sun can mess up the genetic codes in their skin's DNA. And that can trigger skin cancer. Eventually, the killer cells of their immune systems get turned off by the same rays and skin tumors begin to grow.

Think of it this way, says Edward De Fabo, Ph.D., a research photobiologist at George Washington University Medical Center, "You go out into the sunshine. You get some sun on your skin and – even if you tan – the DNA is going to absorb some of those rays. So now you're running the risk of altering those molecules. And as soon as you do that, if they're altered sufficiently so the cells look different to the immune system, then the immune system is going to think these cells are foreign.

"If they think that your skin cells are foreign, then they're going to stimulate an 'up' response

– that is, your immune system's alarm is going to go off.

"But you have to have a way to 'down' modulate that effect," says Dr. De Fabo, "because, after all, you don't want a sort of uncontrolled attack against your own skin. So the immune system then switches on another kind of down-modulating cell – a suppressor cell – and this dampens the up signal so things go back into a state of balance."

Too much sunshine sends your immune system on a roller coaster ride.

YOUR SKIN'S CHEMICAL ANTENNA

How does the immune system activate your down signal? "My wife and colleague, Frances Noonan, Ph.D., and I discovered that a unique molecule sits on the surface of the skin like an antenna. It absorbs the sun's rays and then does a little flip-flop. It changes itself three dimensionally. And, like a light switch, it switches on the suppressor cells."

Usually, says Dr. De Fabo, that's enough to keep your immune system from attacking your skin as you frolic on the beach. But there is a price.

A malignant cell in the skin can go unnoticed.

"Let's say you just get a little bit too much UVB [the harmful part of sunlight]," says Dr. De Fabo. "Then one of your skin cells – these are very sensitive to sunlight – becomes malignant. Now think of that malignant cell as being sort of hidden among all the sun-damaged cells. If the suppressor cells shut down the attack against the sun-damaged cells, they may inadvertently shut down the attack against that transformed malignant cell, as well. You accidentally end up protecting a skin tumor."

LEARN TO PROTECT YOUR IMMUNE SYSTEM

You may also inadvertently end up suppressing other parts of your immune system.

"These UVB rays have been shown to be able to cause systemic immune suppression," confirms Dr. De Fabo, at least in the lab. In one study, for example, Australian researchers exposed 12 people to 30 minutes of a sunlamp on 12 consecutive days. Despite a sunscreen, the researchers reported, the natural killer cells normally deployed by the participants' immune systems against an invader were sharply reduced. And they stayed reduced for 21 days after exposure.

There is a very intricate balance between sunlight and the immune system.

What does this mean? "What we probably have is a very intricate balance between sunlight and the immune system," says Dr. De Fabo. "And UVB clearly has an effect on the immune system. So I think the message that needs to be gotten across is to use some common sense. If you're fair and you burn and you don't tan very well and you spend an awful lot of time outdoors, you're probably gonna be activating your immune system beyond what it can normally take. So just be a little more prudent in your exposure."

John M. Douglass, M.D., a Los Angeles internist who has noticed an increased incidence of herpes in people who get lots of sun, agrees. "Stay out of the sun between 10:00 A.M. and 4:00 P.M.," advises Dr. Douglass, and when you're outside, head for the shade as much as possible.

The National Center for Health Statistics also recommends that outdoor workers wear sunscreens, wide-brimmed hats, and wraparound sunglasses, while others suggest that people with untanned skin should forget the sunscreens and reach for a sunblock.

As for x-rays and other types of ionizing radiation, keep in mind that these forms are far more intense – more energetic, scientists like to say – than radiation produced by sunlight. With ionizing radiation, says Dr. De Fabo, the DNA in your skin cells is not just altered, it's actually broken into a zillion tiny pieces. So reduce your exposure to it as much as possible.

One way is to limit your x-rays in hospital and dental offices. Ask your dentist if an x-ray is actually necessary to confirm his diagnosis or "just routine." Make sure you're covered by a lead shield and check to see that any dental x-ray machine pointed at you has an 8-inch-long, lead-lined attachment that limits the width of the radiating beam.

Limit your exposure to x-rays, which are far more intense in their effects than sunlight.

Another way to avoid radiation is to be aware of potential sources in your environment. Airport inspection systems and television sets are fairly significant sources, as is the equipment in mobile x-ray units at health fairs. Mass screening programs are wonderful in theory, doctors say, but the equipment involved undergoes such rough handling that you may be exposed to more radiation than you should be.

What's the bottom line? Protect your immune system from radiation. Then it can protect you.

36

RASHES:
AN ITCHY ISSUE

Itch?

If it's any consolation, you're not alone. Rashes and their accompanying itch are the common lot. We all itch at one time or another. Picture millions of people around the earth sighing with the collective satisfaction of a good scratch, and you won't be too far from wrong.

Lay the blame for itch on your immune system.

Whether those red eruptions polka-dotting your skin are caused by mosquito bites, poison ivy, contact dermatitis, or food allergy, you really have but one culprit to pin the blame on. The finger points directly to your immune system.

Your skin is, after all, an immune system organ, your personal barrier against the outside world. Your skin contains, among other things, mast cells. Mast cells play a key role in making some people's lives miserable. When stimulated by allergens, mast cells release histamines and other inflammation-causing chemicals.

Any kind of inflammation – including a rash – is an immune system response. The skin releases chemicals sounding the alarm that *something* is irritating it and all kinds of immune cells rush to the rescue. When enough of them collect under the skin, they cause redness and swelling. If you want to stop the rash, you have to eliminate all those irritating "somethings" from your life. That can prove to be quite a trick.

BORN TO RASH

Atopic dermatitis (you probably call it eczema) affects up to 10 percent of all children, according to Hugh Sampson, M.D., associate professor of pediatrics at Johns Hopkins University. But it isn't limited to children. Many adults continue the daily battle against the stubborn rash that is more common in industrialized societies, due in part to our airtight buildings. It also tends to run in families. If your parents have sensitive skin that breaks out at the least provocation, you probably do, too.

Atopic dermatitis is sometimes called "the itch that rashes," because if you can keep from scratching it (you can *try*), the rash won't develop. In both children and adults, the treatment consists in large part of controlling the itching, says Dr. Sampson.

Everyone's skin is different, but here are a number of tips that Dr. Sampson recommends to his patients.

Avoid irritants. Use mild soaps such as Neutrogena, oatmeal, or Dove. Try adding Alpha-Keri lotion to the bath water 5 minutes before getting out of the tub. Apply moisturizing cream immediately after drying off.

Keep cool. Keeping the skin cool and dry helps. Install air conditioning in the bedroom.

Don't sweat. Sweating just makes it worse. "Heat, humidity, exercise, stress, and anxiety are all things that make you sweat, and sweat can trigger itching in a patient with atopic dermatitis," Dr. Sampson warns. Exercise that produces prolonged sweating can be especially troublesome. You might get away with it if you take a cool shower immediately afterward. Or, better yet, try swimming.

Consider food allergies. The most common food allergies in children are eggs, peanuts, and milk. Next come soy products, wheat, and

Atopic dermatitis plagues many children and some adults.

Use mild soaps, stay cool, and don't sweat.

fish. "Those together make up 90 percent of the reactions we see," says Dr. Sampson.

If you suspect a food allergy, you'll need the help of a specialist to determine what foods you should avoid.

LOOK, BUT DON'T TOUCH

After all is said and done, the most common cause of rashes is not something that you eat. It's more likely to be something that you touch, says skin allergy specialist Leonard Grayson, M.D., clinical associate at Southern Illinois University Medical School.

Contact dermatitis is public enemy number one when it comes to rash.

Contact dermatitis is public enemy number one when it comes to rash. You brush up against one of those irritating "somethings" that surround us and, bang, you break out in a rash. The itching begins.

Before we move on to a list of the most common offending "somethings" that cause contact dermatitis, let's take a closer look at that irritating itch. Ever wonder what an itch is exactly?

"There are two theories about that," explains Dr. Grayson. "One is that the terminal pain fibers get a subliminal stimulation, so instead of pain, you feel itch. There are no itch fibers as such. The other theory is that a substance called substance P is released that causes itching."

Itching is so irritating that most people prefer pain.

The sensations of pain and itching ride the same nerve pathways to your brain, according to Dr. Sampson. Itching is so darned irritating that most of us would rather have a little pain instead. That's why we scratch.

But you're probably more interested in how to *stop* itching rather than in why you itch.

POISON IVY

You enjoyed that camping trip – the savory aroma of frying bacon beckoning you to breakfast, the hike through the misty green woods, the

pretty plants – but you're not enjoying the sou-
venirs of the trip – the red rash, the itch, the
itch, the *ITCH.*

Remember those pretty plants? If you make
the mistake of being attracted to the autumn
blaze of poison ivy or poison oak, the memory
of your camping trip will stay with you in very
real ways.

It's the most common allergy of all. More
people react to urushiol – the clear, gummy oil
that runs through the resin canals of poison oak,
ivy, and sumac – than to any other substance on
the face of the earth.

Half the population is "clinically sensitive"
– that means they're sure to react after they
come into contact with one of the plants. Another
35 percent of the population will react only to
higher concentrations or longer exposures. A
scant 15 percent are so tolerant they could rub
it all over themselves without a reaction.

Fully half the population is sensitive to poison ivy.

Oddly enough, people with food, drug, mold,
or pollen allergies are likely to be members of
that tolerant group. The people who react to
the plants generally *don't* have a history of those
kinds of allergies, says William Epstein, M.D.,
professor of dermatology at the University of
California, San Francisco. But people who react
to things that touch their skin (contact allergies) are another story. They are the *prime* can-
didates for an allergic reaction to poison oak,
ivy, or sumac.

"Most people already know if they're sensitive or not from previous exposure," explains
Dr. Epstein. For those who have reacted in the
past, avoidance is the best advice. But learning
just what to avoid is a little trickier than boy
scout manuals would have you believe.

The best way to deal with poison ivy is to avoid it entirely.

"These plants vary greatly in size and shape
in different parts of the country," warns Dr. Epstein,
"so pictures in books are often no help at all.
Generally, the Rockies form the dividing line
that separates East Coast poison ivy from West

Coast poison oak. But down in Texas there is a hybrid with characteristics of both plants. If you want to avoid exposure, you've got to find out what these plants look like in your area. The local public health department should be able to supply that information."

POISON, POISON EVERYWHERE

The urushiol oil in these plants is incredibly concentrated and never dormant. It's active even in the dead of winter and commonly causes reactions in skiers and people who unknowingly gather the plants' twigs for kindling. Urushiol runs through the leaves, roots, vines – "every part of the plant but the flowers," explains Dr. Epstein, who says that's why the honey made by bees from these flowers isn't allergenic. ("But it tastes bitter and terrible," he adds.)

Some of these flowers are truly beautiful – an attraction that accounts for a good number of California poison oak cases. Dr. Epstein himself has visited homes where the fresh-cut flowers were on display and advised the gatherers to "call him in the morning" – since the symptoms of this allergy often come on so slowly that most people won't even notice it for several days.

Calamine lotion is still the best treatment.

When those symptoms first begin to appear, "it looks like a flea bite," says Dr. Epstein. "The area becomes red and itchy after 48 hours and the blisters appear a few days later. Calamine lotion, available at any drugstore, is the best treatment."

Extremely sensitive people – some 10 to 15 percent of those who react – are a different story. "It's one of the few true emergencies in dermatology," says Dr. Epstein. "They'll get red, itchy, and start to swell up within 4 to 12 hours. By the next day, their eyes can be swollen shut. The blisters are there within 24 hours. These people must get to a hospital for a shot of corticosteroids. If they get the shot fast enough and get a large enough dosage of a medication such as prednisone, we can actually stop the swelling and make them comfortable."

THE GIFT THAT GOES ON GIVING

The initial exposure – touching, or walking through the plants – is only the beginning of the problem. Since most symptoms don't develop immediately, people don't think to wash the affected areas – and the invisible oil then gets on everything with which they come in contact. Dr. Epstein recalls one patient who touched the plants and then drove home: "He kept picking it up for weeks from the steering wheel of his car!"

If you develop symptoms and connect them with poison oak or ivy, Dr. Epstein says to "go back and wash *everything* you touched." You don't even need soap – plain water will do the trick. In fact, an immediate wash may end the problem before the reaction starts.

"If you think you've been exposed while picnicking, hiking, gardening, golfing, or hunting, take a dip in a stream or soak yourself with a hose," says Dr. Epstein. "You can also use rubbing alcohol. In fact, the best possible treatment would be alcohol followed by water. In any case, don't use a washrag. The cloth will only pick it up and spread it around.

"But remember, this works only if you wash right away. If you wait until you get home, it may be too late," cautions Dr. Epstein.

> If people don't wash the affected areas, the oil from the plant gets on everything.

CONTACT DERMATITIS

Poison ivy is not the only game in town. Plenty of other substances can get under your skin. There's a whole plethora of offenders – everything from your aunt's heirloom ring that leaves a rashy ring around your finger to that fragrant lipstick that drools a red rash down your chin.

If your skin is sensitive, you need to be a

> Plenty of other substances can cause allergic reaction.

real detective to ferret out what's bugging you. Here are some hints. These leading causes of allergic skin reactions are provided by Robert Adams, M.D., clinical professor of dermatology at Stanford University. He also has a number of suggestions on how to avoid these substances, which seem to be all over the place.

Nickel. Almost anything made of metal may contain some nickel, but jewelry, buttons, clasps, and other objects that stay in contact with the skin for extended periods of time are the cause of most reactions.

For alternatives, select aluminum, stainless steel (its nickel content is high, but its chemical makeup is such that the nickel can't reach the skin), and 18-carat gold. White gold releases nickel and is *not* a good substitute.

Some nickel-sensitive people have had their hand symptoms improve when they changed to a diet low in nickel. Here are the guidelines.

- Avoid these foods high in nickel: all canned foods and all foods cooked in nickel-plated utensils, herring, oysters, asparagus, beans, mushrooms, onions, corn, spinach, peas, tomatoes, whole grain flour, pears, rhubarb, tea, cocoa, chocolate, and baking powder.
- These foods are permitted without limit: all other fish, meats, poultry, eggs, dairy products, and margarine.
- These foods are permitted in moderation: potatoes (one small spud per day), cauliflower, cabbage, carrots, cucumbers, lettuce, rice, refined flour, fresh fruit, jams and jellies, coffee, beer, and wine.

Note: Many cases of nickel allergy begin when ears are pierced and nickel-containing earrings are inserted.

Neomycin. The most common topical (applied to the skin) antibiotic is also one of the most common topical allergens. People sensi-

Almost anything made of metal may contain some nickel.

Avoid foods high in nickel.

The most common topical antibiotic is one of the most common topical allergens.

tive to this medication may also react to these other antibiotics: gentamicin, streptomycin, kanamycin, and framycetin. Although it isn't closely related to neomycin, bacitracin has also caused serious reactions in sensitive individuals and is not recommended as a substitute.

For an alternative, request erythromycin, which is not a known cause of allergy problems. However, Akne-mycin, a popular erythromycin ointment, contains a fragrance that may cause problems.

Your best bet is to ask your local pharmacy to prepare erythromycin that's free of fragrance. They can prepare it by mixing a powdered form of the antibiotic in a small amount of mineral oil with petrolatum to make an ointment.

Quaternium-15. This chemical keeps germs from growing in cosmetics, but it is a leading cause of contact allergy for many women. It also releases small amounts of formaldehyde that may cause people who are allergic to that substance to react as well. The only alternative here is to read labels and avoid all cosmetics that contain this preservative.

Chemicals in cosmetics and rubber goods can cause problems.

MBT and Thiuram mix. These chemical additives are the major causes of contact allergy to such rubber goods as gloves, shoes, aprons – even rubber bands and balloons.

People who are allergic to one of these chemicals (known as accelerators) are frequently sensitive to others as well. The best option is to avoid rubber goods in favor of articles made with polyvinyl chloride (PVC), polyvinyl acetate, polyethylene, or silicone.

Watch out for boxer shorts with elastic waistbands, condoms (note that the brands made with animal products rather than latex do *not* stop the AIDS virus), swim goggles, and shoes made with rubber.

Mercapto mix. The most commonly used epoxy resin in industry is the leading cause of epoxy allergy. It's used in dental materials, elec-

Epoxy and balsam peru are problems for sensitive people.

tronic parts, wall surfaces, panels, and paints, and is added to cements and mortar.

Balsam peru. This is also called Indian balsam, China oil, or Surinam balsam. Although used as a flavoring, especially in chocolate, and as an ingredient in cough drops and syrups, balsam peru causes the most problems when added as a fragrance. People with prolonged skin problems due to an allergy to this substance may benefit from avoiding foods suspected of containing balsam peru: citrus juices and other products containing citrus peel, such as marmalade, baked goods, cocktails, candy, and chewing gum; products that are flavored with essences or perfumed, such as scented teas and tobaccos; ice cream; colas and other flavored soft drinks; and spices such as cinnamon, cloves, vanilla, and curry (this includes products made with those spices, such as catsup, chili, pickled products, baked goods, pâté, and vermouth).

A number of medical preparations also contain balsam peru, including many forms of cough medicines and lozenges; eugenol, used by dentists as a topical antiseptic and painkiller; and many hemorrhoidal preparations.

For most people with this allergy, fragrance-free cosmetics from Clinique, Almay, or Allercreme shouldn't cause a problem. Read labels carefully.

Formaldehyde. Although many people are concerned about inhalation of this material, the most common reactions come from skin contact. Formaldehyde is present in small amounts in many substances, including cosmetics, topical medications, leather goods, photographic chemicals, and cigarette smoke.

Some shampoos contain formaldehyde, but these are believed to cause problems only for those with the most extreme sensitivity, since they remain in contact with the scalp for so short a period of time.

Another form of the chemical, known as

Although many people are concerned about inhaling formaldehyde, the most common reactions come from skin contact.

paraformaldehyde, is found in fungicides, bactericides, disinfectants, adhesives, gelatin, and some contraceptive creams and foot powders.

Formaldehyde is also used in some dry-cleaning formulas, as well as in dyes and textiles, especially permanent-press fabrics. But problems with formaldehyde in clothing and other fabrics now occur much less frequently than in the past. You can remove the formaldehyde that is released from treated fabrics by adding a cupful or two of powdered milk (yes, milk) to the detergent in the wash water for two or three washings in a row. This works especially well for newly purchased permanent-press fabrics such as sheets, pillowcases, shirts, and blouses.

Untreated, unfinished cotton fibers, such as blue jeans, are believed to be free of all allergenic materials, including formaldehyde. Untreated nylon is also thought to be safe. Silk, linen, and Ultrasuede (a polyester) are also considered safe, as are products that have been sized, Sanforized, or mercerized.

Phenylenediamine. Formerly a problem when used in fur and textile dyes, almost all cases of sensitivity to this substance are now caused by its presence in permanent and semi-permanent hair dyes. Even those permanent dyes without Phenylenediamine contain a related chemical that can cause problems.

Almost all cases of sensitivity to phenylenediamine are caused by its presence in hair dyes.

Hair dyes get things started, but once the allergy develops, those affected may also react to aniline and azo dyes (used in foods, cosmetics, and medications), PABA (used in many sunscreen lotions), local anesthetics such as benzocaine and procaine, and many other substances – including rubber, which can contain a form of the chemical as an ingredient.

Temporary hair tints cause the fewest problems. Tints labeled "semipermanent" contain related chemicals but are much less likely to cause a reaction than permanent dyes. Henna is considered safe.

Wool alcohols. These are also called lanolin alcohols, and yes, these products actually do come from sheep. They're used primarily in cosmetics and topical medications but can also be found in leather, shoe polishes, lubricants, waxes, and soaps. Contact allergy problems only seem to develop when these ingredients are present in concentrations greater than 3 percent.

Read labels to avoid lanolin in cosmetics.

For cosmetics, read labels. Lanolin-sensitive individuals should always mention this problem to doctors and pharmacists.

Benzocaine. This topical painkiller is not believed to be a strong sensitizer in itself, but it often becomes an allergy problem when used on already-irritated skin.

Substitution is no problem because there are a number of alternate products. Relief of itching is better accomplished by treating the dermatitis with conventional methods, including topical steroid creams. Read labels carefully.

Thimerosal. This is also called Merthiolate or sodium ethylmercurithiosalicylate. Although it's used as a preservative in vaccines as well as in nasal and eye medications (including contact lens solutions), many of the people allergic to this substance were originally sensitized by a skinned knee. Tincture of Merthiolate, that red stuff our mothers used to swab over cuts and scrapes when we were kids, contains the component of the chemical that is believed to cause allergic reactions.

In vaccines, make sure that phenol has been used as the preservative. As an antiseptic, use Betadine skin cleanser or Hibiclens (chlorohexidine). Eye medications that contain chiorobautanol or benzalkonium chloride are good substitutes.

For contact lens solutions, look for sterile saline preparations such as Unisol Preservative-free Saline Solution and Lens Plus.

37

RELAXATION: SOOTHING YOUR IMMUNE SYSTEM

You've got to take the exam. You pick up your pencil, flip open the test book, and stare at the instructions in bold type. None of them make any sense. You grip your pencil, move the test closer, and try to focus your mind. Don't panic, you say to yourself. You can do it.

And you do. You take the exam, turn in your test, and walk out of the room. You're exhausted, but riding a high that just won't quit. That is, until you sneeze.

Sneeze? Where did that come from? You must be getting a cold. But your resistance is usually so good. How come you got the virus? How come your body didn't just fight it off?

Suprisingly, the answer may be your exam. Or at least the worry and stress you experienced in the weeks just before it.

In a striking study at the Ohio State University College of Medicine, for example, 75 first-year medical students had blood samples taken a month before their final exams and during the first day of testing. The results, measured by laboratory analysis, indicated that even the relatively minor stress of an exam wiped out nearly 10 percent of the natural killer cells patrolling their bodies.

And a second study at Ohio State – again using first-year medical students – indicated that the anxiety levels during exams taken by these

Anxiety can cut your infection fighters by *half*.

soon-to-be doctors cut the number of infection-fighting helper T-cells by just about *half.* The normal percentage of helper T's in the students' blood should have been between 34 and 54 percent, the researchers reported. It wasn't. In blood taken after a three-day exam, it was less than 20 percent.

Chronic stress not only makes you more vulnerable to infection, at the same time it cuts your defensive forces by 41 percent.

Unfortunately, chronic stress – as opposed to the situational stress of an exam – apparently produces the same result. In a third Ohio State study – this one of 34 people who had family members with Alzheimer's disease who were living at home – blood samples revealed that the caregivers were roughly 41 percent more susceptible to viral infections than people who did not care for an ailing relative. And, while the caregivers were more susceptible to infection, the helper T's available to fight the infection *dropped* by 37 percent.

Not only were the caregivers more susceptible to infection, the researchers concluded, they were also less able to fight when attacked.

HOW DOES STRESS SUPPRESS?

Relaxation seems to counter the negative chemicals produced by stress.

How does stress suppress your immune system? Scientists suspect that it triggers "fight-or-flight" chemicals – such as steroids and corticosteroids from the adrenal glands – which in turn suppress the immune system. Distress also causes a release of vasopressin, a hormone that slows antibody movement – further lowering your immune protection. Whatever chemical reaction stress triggers, relaxing seems to counter it. It's almost as though relaxation releases a new set of chemicals that actually neutralize the ones released by stress.

One study indicates that a relaxation technique can increase your helper T-cells by 38 percent.

In another study at Ohio State, for example, researchers taught students a mixed bag of relaxation techniques and suggested that they practice the techniques outside of class. The result?

Students who learned how to relax increased the number of helper T-cells circulating in their blood by 38 percent. And the more they actually practiced the techniques they learned, the more helper T's reported for duty.

In another study, the Ohio State researchers used 45 men and women between the ages of 60 and 88 to show that relaxation exercises three times a week for a month increased natural killer cell activity by roughly 18 percent and *de*creased the study participants' susceptibility to viral invaders.

Yet another study – this one at Albright College in Pennsylvania – tested saliva samples from a group of volunteers both before and after a variety of relaxation techniques were practiced. The increased levels of immunoglobulin A – an antibody stationed at the openings of your body – indicate that no matter which way you choose to relax, 20 minutes of mentally getting away from it all will clearly boost your immune system.

LEARN TO RELAX

The evidence that relaxation enhances immune function seems overwhelming. Equally evident seems the fact that how you get yourself into a relaxed state probably doesn't matter. But the method that most researchers seem to use is Progressive Muscle Relaxation, a technique in which you focus on the naturally existing tension in a group of muscles and then consciously release it.

Focus on the naturally existing tension in a group of muscles, then consciously release it.

Want to try it? The best way to begin a relaxation exercise is to find a quiet place away from any distractions, loosen your clothing, and snuggle your body into a comfortable chair or couch, explains Martin L. Rossman, M.D., a clinical associate at the University of California, San Francisco.

Take a couple of deep breaths, advises Dr. Rossman, breathing in deeply, and exhaling all your stress as you expel the air. Then, beginning with one of your feet, notice how the tension feels in that particular appendage and let the tension go. Just let it flow away. Repeat the exercise with your other foot, then move progressively higher – through your calves, thighs, buttocks, back, shoulders, arms, neck – until, finally, even your scalp is relaxed. Then luxuriate in the blissful feeling of total body relaxation.

Twenty minutes twice a day will boost your immune power, one doctor says.

The entire exercise should take you about 20 to 25 minutes, says Dr. Rossman, so make sure you have enough time set aside to enjoy it. If you're trying to boost your immune system, he suggests, you should do the exercise twice a day.

Another way to learn how to relax is with biofeedback. Researchers at North Texas State University, for example, hooked a group of students up to machines that measured such biological responses as muscle tone and skin temperature. And, as the students learned to relate the instruments' measurements to a particular level of relaxation, the study reveals that they also learned to deepen their state of relaxation. The result was an increase in the number of their phagocytes – scavenger cells that eat invading microbes – by 37 percent.

Learn a technique and use it to help your immune system.

Impressive statistics aside, what does this information mean to you? In a sense, it means you have some control – control over even the involuntary functions of your body. It means that when you're faced with a difficult, worrisome time in your life, you can help to protect yourself from becoming ill. You can practice a relaxation technique to soothe your nerves and also help bolster the immune system. Select the technique that you like best, learn it, then make a habit of using it when the going gets tough.

38

RHEUMATIC FEVER:
AN ATTACK ON THE HEART

Let a known child abuser out of jail and just watch how parents close ranks and become protective of their little ones.

An old familiar face, hidden away for the past two decades, is showing up once again in classrooms and on playgrounds. And it's time to sound the alert. This child abuser is particularly treacherous. It sneaks in disguised as an ordinary strep throat, but then it takes a nasty turn that can lead to lifelong heart damage, even death.

The threat is rheumatic fever, an autoimmune nightmare. The disease was so prevalent at the turn of the century that entire hospitals were devoted to the care of children suffering from it. Rheumatic fever strikes young adults as well as children and used to be such a problem in military barracks that new recruits were routinely given antibiotics to protect them during basic training.

Rheumatic fever was prevalent at the turn of the century.

Then the damaging disease all but disappeared, at least in the United States. Recent years have seen only 1 case per 100,000 school-age children. Those few cases tended to be among poorer, urban, primarily black families because *Streptococcus pyogenes,* the group A streptococcus bacteria responsible for rheumatic fever, thrives in overcrowded conditions, according to Alan Bisno, M.D., professor of medicine at the University of Miami School of Medicine.

OLD ENEMY, NEW GUISE

Recent outbreaks have been reported in Utah, Pennsylvania, and Ohio.

Recent outbreaks of rheumatic fever reported in Salt Lake City, Utah; Pittsburgh, Pennsylvania; and Akron and Columbus, Ohio, have been primarily among white, middle-class families living in suburban or rural areas. These surprising outbreaks mean that *Streptococcus pyogenes* is not behaving the way it usually does. Scientists think a particularly virulent strain of the strep bacteria may be responsible.

Virulent or not, the bacteria haven't changed the way they go about making sick children sicker.

Rheumatic fever is an auto-immune disease that can follow strep throat.

"The most prevalent theory is that there are a lot of similarities between certain structures in the group A streptococcus and tissues in the human heart. The body is trying to make an immune response against the streptococcus, but it inadvertently makes an immune response against human connective tissues in the joints and the heart," says Dr. Bisno.

When you get a strep throat, your immune system does what it's supposed to do. It recognizes strep bacteria as enemies and it manufactures antibodies to zap the invaders. But then confusion reigns. Theory holds that, to those antibodies that are tailor-made to attack strep, joints and heart tissue look awfully familiar. They look, in theory, just like those strep bacteria that have no business being in your body. Wham, the antibodies apparently hone in on the joints and the heart, trying to drive the "enemy invaders" right out of the body. The result is one very sick child.

When the antibodies attack the joints, they appear to produce a sort of migratory arthritis in which pain and inflammation seem to move from one area of the body to another. When they attack the heart, permanent damage may result. Millions of adults around the world suffer from faulty heart valves as a result of a childhood bout with rheumatic fever. The disease is still prevalent in underdeveloped countries.

BLOCK THAT PUNCH

Not every strep throat leads to rheumatic fever. And not every case of rheumatic fever leads to damaging heart disease. But who wants to take a chance?

A child with strep throat will have pain on swallowing, a fever, and perhaps tender lymph nodes at the angles of the jaws, or a rash.

"If such symptoms occur, you should definitely not assume that it's nothing to worry about," says Dr. Bisno. "You should contact your pediatrician."

Young adults, too, have reason to be concerned about such symptoms, but the risk of rheumatic fever is not as great.

A doctor will take a throat culture to determine whether the sore throat is indeed a strep throat, and if it is, will prescribe antibiotics to knock it out before rheumatic fever can develop.

A child with strep throat must visit a doctor.

39

RHEUMATOID ARTHRITIS: AN AUTOIMMUNE MYSTERY

Leslie, 26, is a pert and perky redhead who often stars in local theater productions, sings in the church choir, and races stock cars. But today high-energy Leslie has taken to her bed. She has chills and fever, she's sweating, and she feels exhausted.

A casual observer might guess she has the flu. But Leslie knows she doesn't have the flu because, in addition to her whole-body symptoms, her joints are red and hot, and she is developing nodules on her elbows. She recognizes this as another cycle in a round of rheumatoid arthritis (RA), a disease that attacks the entire body as well as the joints.

The causes of RA are still a mystery, but it is probably an autoimmune disease.

The disease is chronic and can be disfiguring. The finest medical minds in the world can't figure out exactly what causes it, but their best guess is that it is an autoimmune disease, that is, a disease in which the body's immune system attacks its own tissue.

FAILURE OF RECOGNITION

It's as if Leslie's immune system looked in a mirror and asked, "Who's that?" Her immune system fails at a crucial task – self-recognition – and instead of protecting its own body against disease, literally attacks it with the ferocity it should save for germs.

264

The true nature of RA is a mystery. "It doesn't take us long to get to areas of our ignorance," says David Wofsy, M.D., assistant professor of medicine at the University of California, San Francisco. "No one really knows what happens in rheumatoid arthritis, although it's certain there are antibodies against the host."

The sherlocks investigating RA have devised three main theories, Dr. Wofsy says. One is that the antibodies attack with no apparent cause. Another theory is that something – a virus, perhaps – damages the synovial membrane that surrounds and lubricates the joint. The virus alters the synovial membrane's appearance so the antibodies don't recognize it as part of the body and go on the offensive. Yet another scenario suggests that molecules on a virus or toxin so closely resemble host molecules that the immune response to the foreign substance doesn't stop there but goes right on to attack the body.

No one knows what causes antibodies to attack.

THE STAGES OF RA

Untreated – and sometimes even treated – rheumatoid arthritis has four stages.

- The rheumatoid factor (RF) assaults the synovial membrane, causing chronic inflammation and thickening. RF is made up of antibodies produced by B-cells. Surprisingly, it is apparently a normal component of the immune system from birth and may provide a beneficial edge to the developing immune system. Nobody knows why it sometimes turns and attacks the body.
- In stage two, a layer of tissue called pannus is formed. With time, it erodes and destroys the cartilage and eventually the bone and parts of the muscles that control the joint.

RA begins with inflammation and progresses to tissue damage.

- The joint begins to lose mobility because tough fibers invade the pannus.
- Mobility is further lessened as this fibrous tissue becomes calcified.

RA generally attacks the hands and wrists, but it can also hit the knees, the balls of the feet, or the spine.

Even your heart doesn't escape RA.

But RA doesn't limit itself to joints. It goes after the entire body, and without treatment it can be life threatening. Muscles, bones, and skin near the affected joints atrophy. Nodules form beneath the skin, especially on the elbows. The membrane encasing the heart and lungs can become inflamed, the spleen can enlarge, and anemia can develop. Flulike symptoms are common.

About 20 percent of those who get RA recover completely. In about 60 percent the disease flares up and dies down over the years. Irreversible joint damage afflicts the remainder. The good news is that RA eventually burns itself out. Although most RA sufferers are in the prime of life, the disease doesn't discriminate based on age.

RA strikes equal numbers of women and men, but three times as many women get symptoms severe enough to need medical attention. Symptoms, however, often decline or even disappear during pregnancy. This remarkable remission leads researchers to think hormones could have something to do with RA, but there's no conclusive evidence.

With widely varying success, other researchers have linked RA's cause or symptoms to allergy, heredity, infections, emotional states, copper, physical injuries, diet, even the weather. And each theory has led to a matching therapy that is also more or less successful – and a huge host of scams designed for the desperate.

Still, despite enormous amounts of time and money and some of the best brains in science, the mystery persists. All doctors can do is try to treat the symptoms.

OLD TOOLS, NEW USES

The key to treatment of rheumatoid arthritis – indeed, any autoimmune disease – is immunosuppressive therapy. Doctors try to suppress the immune system to the point where the symptoms diminish, without going so far that you become susceptible to infection. This treatment is the same kind of high-wire act most vividly seen in organ transplantation, when the immune system works its little antibodies off trying to kill the transplanted organ.

The key to pain relief is to suppress your immune system.

With RA, inflammation is the enemy. Inflammation is the most visible sign of an active immune system – the redness and soreness surrounding a cut show that your white blood cells are fighting and killing germs. But in RA, inflammation is the destroyer of healthy and essential cells.

The RA mystery extends to the drugs used to treat it. Even the workings of aspirin and ibuprofen haven't been completely deciphered. But what is really important is that we know that these drugs work.

"The first line of attack in rheumatoid arthritis is aspirin and aspirinlike drugs," Dr. Wofsy says. Choline magnesium trisalicylate and enteric-coated or buffered aspirin are relatively safe and powerful painkillers and anti-inflammatory drugs and "are sufficient for many people." So effective are these drugs that maybe one-quarter of people with RA recover completely with this relatively simple treatment.

Aspirin and aspirinlike drugs cure 25 percent of those with RA.

The nonsteroidal anti-inflammatory drugs, the NSAIDs, are also good painkillers and anti-inflammatories, but they are usually no better than aspirin. Some have serious side effects. The NSAIDs include phenylbutazone (such as Azolid), ibuprofen (such as Advil), and naproxen (such as Naprosyn).

On the next rung of the treatment ladder are the corticosteroids, potent anti-inflammatory hormones. They are intended for more severe cases, and their adverse side effects can also be more severe. They increase susceptibility to infection and delay wound healing. They have many other serious side effects, including dependency.

Researchers are finding new ways to use "old" drugs.

"Then there are drugs for which the mechanism of how they work is *completely* unknown," Dr. Wofsy says. "Back to the future" is the key phrase here; researchers have found new ways to use "old" drugs.

Gold was originally used to treat tuberculosis, he says, but in RA it was found to fight inflammation and induce remission. Remission-inducing chloroquine began as an antimalarial drug. Methotrexate suppresses the immune system by killing white blood cells, and thus it was originally used to treat leukemia before researchers stumbled on it as an RA therapy. Cyclosporine, another immune suppressant, is used in organ transplants. Penicillamine was first used to treat a rare disease of copper metabolism and is now an RA treatment of last resort.

Side effects are a problem with arthritis drugs.

"These drugs all have four things in common," Dr. Wofsy says. "We don't know how they work. They all reduce inflammation. They're severely toxic – one-third of rheumatoid arthritis patients get significant unpleasant side effects. And they don't work in everybody."

THE CASE FOR FOOD

Diets, whether of food avoidance (based on the food allergy theory) or additions, are a common alternative therapy, but here again it's not known if they work for any but a very few. "Some have been studied at the biochemical level," Dr. Wofsy says, "and the scientific community is no longer ignoring diet. I hope some-day we'll find the right dietary manipulation for rheumatoid arthritis."

A number of studies, *small* studies, have shown the relationship between diet and RA.

THE FISHY TRUTH

A small percentage of RA sufferers who include fish oil in their diets will find "their disease to be a little less intense," Dr. Wofsy says. "Fish oil appears to have some impact on the inflammatory response. It's demonstrable and real, but not great." In fact, a report in the British medical journal *Lancet* says that if fish oil were a new anti-arthritis drug it probably wouldn't be licensed. However, it is not a drug. It is a natural component of food.

Fish oil may reduce your symptoms.

When it *does* work, fish oil – omega-3 – acts on those inflammation-causing neutrophils in the joints, causing them to produce less of a chemical called leukotriene. Leukotriene en-ables the neutrophils to congregate and stick to blood vessel walls, an early step to inflammation.

This positive action doesn't mean *you* should start taking fish-oil capsules. Just as fish oil can keep neutrophils from sticking together, it can stop blood from clotting. If you're taking aspirin, which is also an anticlotting drug, you could be asking for big trouble. Fish oil could alter other components of your immune response. And if you take fish oil in the form of cod-liver oil, you could also get an overdose of vitamin A. Check with your doctor.

Check with your doctor before taking fish oil.

SELENIUM IN SCANDINAVIA

A Danish study of 87 RA patients found all of them to have significantly low levels of selenium. Patients with lower levels had more joints with active arthritis and less joint mobility. The researchers couldn't say whether the low levels had anything to do with diet.

Selenium and vitamin E reduced joint pain and stiffness in one study.

In Norway, doctors gave selenium and vitamin E supplements to ten RA patients. Joint pain and morning stiffness improved significantly in four of the patients.

Should *you* rush out and start taking selenium supplements? Probably not. While selenium is an essential trace mineral, it also can be toxic. In both studies the doctors didn't advise supplements, just more study.

DECIPHERING YOUR DIET

Richard Panush, M.D., chief of clinical immunology, rheumatology, and allergy at the University of Florida College of Medicine, found that many arthritis patients didn't get enough vitamin E and zinc in their diets. These two nutrients play important roles in immunity.

See a registered dietitian recommended by your doctor for nutritional counseling to determine if you're eating a proper diet.

NEITHER CAUSE NOR CURE

Individual foods don't cause the disease.

Dean Metcalfe, M.D., of the National Institute of Allergy and Infectious Diseases, says that a few people's joints will swell in reaction to certain foods. That swelling could make their arthritis symptoms worse. "But once those food symptoms disappear," Dr. Metcalfe says, "these people will *still* have rheumatoid arthritis. Avoiding the problem foods will *not* make their rheumatoid arthritis go away."

He has a strong warning for any RA sufferer seeking to either eat or eliminate foods he or she thinks may influence the disease. "We don't have any reason to believe that foods are an actual *cause* of rheumatoid arthritis," he says. "It would be terrible if people with *any* form of arthritis suddenly stopped following their doctors' instructions and just gave up foods instead."

Diet and supplements may provide a little relief, *if* you don't abandon your doctor's recommended therapy, and *if* you have dietary problems.

MIND OVER JOINTS

Diet, drugs, and many other treatments are all body oriented. While RA may be in your body, your *mind* has power over the pain and progress of the disease. Your mind can help you cope, or it can make things worse.

Your mind has power over the pain.

"It was first thought that there was an inward-directed hostility that kind of mimicked the body attacking itself," says Alex Zautra, Ph.D., director of clinical psychology at Arizona State University. But research has not borne out that theory. "There is no personality syndrome in rheumatoid arthritis. But the illness itself, because of its chronic nature and progressive and predictable course, is likely to lead to adaptations that can be mistaken for personality problems."

The bottom line, says Sanford Roth, M.D., medical director of the Arthritis Center in Phoenix, professor and director of the Aging and Arthritis Program at Arizona State, and a research colleague of Dr. Zautra, is that "it's quite clear that personality itself is quite important, along with stress and adaptation, in responding to the challenges of the disease." Such things as hope, laying on of hands, psychological support, and stress reduction are "the soft stuff of rheumatology, once relegated to lip service," Dr. Roth says. New research shows these have a positive effect on the immune system. There needs to be more research, he acknowledges, "but good clinicians know that depressed, unsupported, acutely, or chronically stressed patients with rheumatoid disease get worse."

Stress aggravates the disease.

A small study cited by Dr. Roth measured what he calls the "hassle index," rating the success of the way RA patients cope with the day-to-day hassles of living. "Those who adapted poorly showed statistically correlated changes in their immune systems as opposed to those people who seemed to find ways to adapt effectively," he says.

INEFFECTIVE COPING

Depression is an example of ineffective coping. Well, who in their right mind *wouldn't* be depressed to be in pain, unable to move freely, so much of the time? Anger is another ineffective way to cope – and also very understandable. And being overly concerned with your physical condition – hypochondria – is a third example. But when you're sick, you're bound to think more intently about your health.

Acceptance is the key to coping.

Some people may become obsessive, Dr. Zautra says, "and be inclined to think, 'There's gotta be an answer.' Acceptance of the illness is the key, but they might indulge in excessive coping, going from one medication to another, looking for the magic bullet or a cure when there is no cure."

DAY BY DAY

RA is tough. Getting through one day can be bad, let alone thinking about the next week or year. "Having a perspective of getting through one day at a time is very valuable," Dr. Zautra says. "Instead of looking at the future as a burden that you'll always have – as people with chronic illnesses often do, feeling helpless and hopeless – it's better to develop the ability to look at life one day at a time. It's better to see even in a single day the variety of experiences available to a person, even a person in pain. There are many other emotions, besides helplessness and hopelessness, that you can feel. And this realization can give you some control over your pain, and make life worth living despite the limitations the disease imposes on you."

MANAGER WANTED

Negative feelings about such a devastating illness are normal. But rather than let them drag you down, let them galvanize you into fighting back. Dr. Zautra points out there are a number of pain management methods a person can learn. "Pain, after all, is a matter of perception," he says. "It comes from the way you think about it." Imagery, relaxation, meditation can all help to deflect your pain. Different methods work for different people.

Let negative feelings galvanize you into fighting back.

There are two basic ways to learn these different methods: Self-instruction, as from a book or tape, and participation in a group or program. Your success depends on the kind of person you are but usually only the most independent can do it on their own. For most, nothing beats the support and companionship of others in the same boat.

NOTHING'S SIMPLE

Some will cope worse than others because of their outlook. But there's more to it than that, Dr. Roth says. "It's complicated because there are really important cofactors. If the person's not getting adequate treatment, if he or she has other diseases, it can affect their health and ability to fight rheumatoid arthritis." And so along with proper medical treatment, there are other things you can do to combat RA.

WORKING OUT THE PAIN

Exercise has been proven to have physical and mental benefits for everyone, but it may be especially good for people with RA. In a Northwestern University study, Paul Caldron, D.O., says, "We were sort of unscientifically impressed that we were able to get patients with rheuma-

Low-impact aerobics seem to help.

toid arthritis to exercise with low-impact aerobics without causing worse inflammation in joints.

"As a matter of fact, we were able to see almost consistent improvement in joint function. And indeed, the thing that surprised us was that we saw decreases in numbers of inflamed joints, and the degree to which they were inflamed and tender. We think that regular and consistent low-impact aerobic exercise does have some sort of modulating effect on the inflammation in the joints. All people with arthritis ought to be able to do some sort of limited exercise. It may even need to be tailored to the individual.

"Our whole philosophy has changed," says Dr. Caldron, a rheumatologist affiliated with the Arizona Arthritis Center. "Instead of having arthritic patients gradually do less and less, we encourage them to do more and more. If you have low-grade, chronic inflammatory changes in the joints, we suspect that regular active exercise will not cause it to get worse and may indeed improve it."

GAIN MORE THAN PAIN RELIEF

Exercise may help even the worst case.

Exercise works even for the very worst cases, no matter how crippling and deformed, Dr. Caldron says. "These people certainly can improve their self-efficacy, their ability to do things on their own, to do more than they once could do, to recapture some activities they once had to give up, without promoting further damage to their joints."

The psychological benefits, he says, "are part of that equation leading to self-efficacy. Not only are these people able to do more, it just sort of spirals. The more that they saw they could do, they would set goals to do more. They'd say, 'Gee, I can do this now, if I work a little harder I'm going to be able to do that again. They develop a can-do attitude through exercise."

That shift in attitude may be caused by an exercise-induced increase in endorphin and enkephalins. These neurotransmitters in the brain, are known as the body's own morphine because of their painkilling and mood-elevating abilities and may be responsible for the so-called runner's high. They have direct and indirect effects on white blood cells.

Consistent exercise may release painkilling neurotransmitters.

"I would bet money that there's certainly a role for endorphins and enkephalins in this sense of self-efficacy," Dr. Caldron says. "People with RA who exercised erratically, who missed sessions, just did not do well. But those who exercised consistently, particularly those who also did some form of aerobic exercise outside the program, uniformly did well. Enkephalin and endorphin levels respond to exercise, and the more consistent exercise you do, the higher base levels of these neurotransmitters you're going to have."

Vigorous, low-impact aerobics includes slow and fast walking, gliding, swaying, sliding, bicycling, and aqua-aerobics. Be sure to consult your doctor first, and have a physical therapist knowledgeable in RA design a program for you.

Stick with it and you can relieve pain, improve your state of mind, reduce the numbers of your joints that are inflamed, and increase your self-reliance and ability to do what you want to. Not a bad way to handle a mystery disease.

THERE'S A TIME FOR EVERYTHIHG

With rheumatoid arthritis, for instance, there's a time to rest. It's when you're having a flare-up. "When a joint is hyper-acutely inflamed," says Dr. Caldron, "obviously you want to put it to rest until the worst part of the inflammation subsides. Rest in itself will decrease the inflammation." Lie on a firm mattress in a good posture, with pillows supporting the joints in a flexed position, and only one pillow under the head.

While you're resting is not only a good time to practice your relaxation skills, it's also a perfect chance to use heat or cold therapy. Since RA also affects the skin, care must be taken to protect it during applications of heat or cold.

Heat helps you relax, improves circulation, and relieves pain. And in conjunction with exercise allows more freedom of joint movement. With heat you have a choice of methods.

Heat in conjunction with exercise allows more joint mobility.

- Dry: therapeutic infrared heat lamps, hot water bottles, or heating pads.
- Moist: hot baths in water not hotter than 102° F; towels dipped in hot water, wrung out, and applied to the joint; or whirlpool baths.
- Diathermy: whether shortwave, ultrasound, or microwave, this type of heat must be applied by an experienced therapist.

Cold is valuable in reducing pain and stiffness. Cold packs can numb swollen joints and quench the fire of inflammation.

Braces, casts, or splints are used to immobilize a joint during a flare-up so it can rest, but you can still get around.

THE FUTURE

The future of arthritis therapy is found in the lab. Scientists at the Mayo Clinic in Rochester, Minnesota, are working on a way to suppress the immune system in specific areas of the body instead of system wide. If it works – and in lab animals it does – it would be a landmark advance in the treatment of many autoimmune diseases.

Subhashis Banerjee, M.D., research associate at the Mayo Clinic's Department of Immunology, says he's basing his research on the theory that the immune system makes antibodies to collagen, the basic connective tissue that holds us all together. There are 15 types of collagen in our bodies, Dr. Banerjee says. "The collagen we think the antibodies attack is a secluded type that usually doesn't come in contact with the immune system unless there is, for instance, an injury. Then the immune system doesn't recognize it as 'self' and attacks it as an antigen."

Dr. Banerjee's research targets T-cells at the point *after* they get the message from macrophages to start cloning, but *before* they actually start proliferating. T-cells use the messenger interleukin-2 to proliferate, and Dr. Banerjee wants to stop that messenger. If the T-cells don't proliferate, then they can't tell B-cells to grow up and start churning out antibodies. So Dr. Banerjee has developed a monoclonal antibody that plugs the socket on the T-cell surface where interleukin-2 normally plugs in.

When the antibody was injected into joints of test animals bred to develop rheumatoid arthritis, "the onset of arthritis was greatly delayed and its severity greatly reduced," Dr. Banerjee says. "We may be able to depopulate T-cells in specific areas, like joints, without the unwanted side effects of system-wide immune suppression." While he has no time frame for trying the therapy on humans, he ventures to guess that the first trials may begin in as soon as five years.

Antibodies may be used to wipe the T-cells out of your joints.

40

SCAMS:
TOO GOOD TO BE TRUE

"If you put a piece of fresh beef inside a vacuum cleaner tube, place the tube over the body, and flip the 'on' switch, you can suck a tumor right out. This works because 'cancerous atoms are magnetic of flesh and blood.' "

Just a few years ago you could buy these instructions through the mail for a mere $25.

And if do-it-yourself cancer cures didn't grab you, you could visit a California practitioner who would – for a fee – hook up electrodes to your body and play "Smoke Gets in Your Eyes." There is no indication whether tumors supposedly cleared out because they didn't like the tune or if the lyrics got to them. But if you wanted to cure arthritis, the electrodes piped in a different tune – "Holiday for Strings."

Quack cures are still with us.

These particular "cures" were denounced as out-and-out fraud in the 1984 U.S. Congressional Report on Quackery. They are no longer available for the desperate patient willing to spend money on anything and everything that holds out even a shred of hope. But for every bogus cure that legal authorities yank out of circulation, new scams stand waiting in the wings.

And if, by chance, you know someone with AIDS, that person can drive south of the border for injections of hydrogen peroxide to oxygenate the blood or take any number of pills and

278

potions with secret ingredients guaranteed to "boost" or "enhance" the immune system.

We might be on the cusp of the 21st century, but medical scams are still alive and well.

QUACKERY LIVES

"Quacks like to get onto the diseases that are complicated, that we currently don't have cures for, that are frustrating, painful, and chronic," says John Renner, M.D., director of community health at Trinity Lutheran Hospital in Kansas City, Missouri, and director of the resource center for the National Council against Health Fraud. "Generally speaking, quacks still like to get desperate people. Anything that creates desperation will do it. And, of course, AIDS is perfect."

AIDS is now attracting its share of quacks.

Americans spend some $25 billion a year on quack remedies, the *Journal of the American Medical Association* has estimated. Phony cancer cures account for $4 to $5 billion of that amount, the article claimed. The 1984 U.S. Congressional Report on Quackery maintained that the elderly alone spend $10 billion a year on bogus cures.

That brings us to the important question of just how to define quackery. No one argues against the inclusion of phony remedies sold by people who know those remedies are bogus, for the single motive of making money.

Yet many mainstream medical professionals also label a number of traditional healing therapies and newer alternative treatments as "quackery" – even when there is evidence suggesting that such approaches may be useful. Some look askance at things like nutrition, acupuncture, and visualization as treatments for chronic disease, for example.

How do you distinguish between alternative therapy and quackery?

"Everything that's ever been new in medicine has been at one time labeled as 'quackery.' We have to make the distinction between 'ineffective' and 'not proved.' There's a lot in medicine that is not proved but very effective," says Christiane Northrup, M.D., assistant clinical professor of obstetrics/gynecology at the University of Vermont School of Medicine and co-president of the American Holistic Medical Association.

BEYOND "SILLY SCIENCE"

More important, how do you protect yourself from quacks?

No one wants to be the victim of an out-and-out quack, but suppose you do want to try an alternative healing treatment. How do you protect yourself from fraud? How can you tell an approach with possible merit from a money-making scam?

Knowing just what kind of treatment you're dealing with is a good place to start.

Dr. Renner, who works with physicians and health professionals around the nation to monitor quackery, has developed his own set of categories to help him understand what is quackery and what isn't.

Dr. Renner's categories are: "folklore," "quackery," "unproven," "experimental," and "proven."

Under "quackery," he includes separate headings for things that are "disproven," such as Laetrile, and remedies that are based on "silly science," such as hydrogen peroxide injections for AIDS.

In the "unproven" category, he puts things that have not yet been tested. "There is some scientific theory behind a lot of things that have not been tested. For AIDS especially, there are a whole bunch of items in this category," says Dr. Renner.

Sometimes Dr. Renner has to work on a case-by-case basis when deciding which category a given treatment goes in. If, for example, a doctor were giving a number of AIDS patients acupuncture, not charging them, and keeping very careful records, Dr. Renner might consider that "experimental." But a health practitioner charging AIDS patients for an acupuncture "cure" would be in another category altogether.

If even medical professionals can quibble over the definitions of "quackery" and "scam," what's the average citizen to do?

Even medical professionals argue over what is quackery.

PROTECTING YOURSELF

If you want to venture off the beaten path for treatment, here are some tips to help you avoid medical rip-offs. These are not meant as the final word but as warning flags for you to activate your common sense and keep your eye on your wallet.

And if you have any doubts about whether a treatment being offered to you is real or bogus, you can always check it with an established medical organization. You might ask the American Diabetes Association about a treatment for diabetes, for example.

If you have any doubts about treatment, check it with an established medical organization.

Here is your set of scam-alert warning flags.

- Be careful if the word "miracle" or "secret" appears.
- Watch out if someone tells you they are the victim of a conspiracy by the American Medical Association, the FDA, the FBI, or some other government body to keep their product off the market.
- Check the person's credentials. Watch out for multiple degrees from strange-sounding or unaccredited institutions or memberships in exotic-sounding

Check credentials and use your common sense.

organizations along the lines of the "World Federation of Scholars Intergalactica."

- Use your common sense. "If everything you've ever heard says up is up, and someone comes along and says up is down or black is white, be careful," says Dr. Renner.
- Don't buy any treatment that purports to cure everything. There is no one potion that will cure arthritis, multiple sclerosis, diabetes, and warts.
- Watch out for products that are going to "boost" or "enhance" your immune system.
- Be careful of people who want to sell you things for both your body and your pets.
- Watch out if someone tries to get you to leave your personal physician or tells you not to trust him or her.
- Beware: No one can guarantee a cure.

There are no guaranteed cures.

Organizations that monitor quackery have a phrase that they like to use: "If it sounds too good to be true, it probably is."

After all is said and done, use your common sense. And when in doubt, check it out.

41

SEXUALLY TRANSMITTED DISEASES: THEY'RE BACK

Venereal disease – that scourge of poets, princes, and paupers alike – was brought to heel by modern antibiotics. For a brief time, it seemed, humankind was free of the worst effects of these diseases. A shot of penicillin cleared up more than the obvious symptoms. It also banished the dread of going blind or insane – which is what happens to someone with untreated syphilis, for example. Sexually transmitted diseases (STDs) fell into line with other communicable diseases – a visit to the doctor, treatment with a miracle drug – and poof! you're cured. We should have suspected that such ancient and awful afflictions would not succumb quite so easily. And they did not.

Penicillin banished the fear.

GONORRHEA

"When it comes to gonorrhea, we don't understand immune mechanisms and how they operate," says James N. Miller, Ph.D., professor of microbiology and immunology at UCLA School of Medicine. Like the influenza virus, the gonococci may disguise themselves so that immune system cells don't recognize them, Dr. Miller says. Nor do they remember the bacteria, enabling your body to build up immunity against the reinfection. And because antibodies don't play any role in immune response to the gonococcus bacteria, there's no constant patrol against the threat.

"For the most part," Dr. Miller says, "the initial infection remains localized in the urethra or cervix. Neutrophils swarm and do battle at the site, and if there aren't enough bacteria, the disease won't occur."

Seventy to 90 percent of women infected with gonorrhea have no symptoms.

But if the bacteria do prevail, a severe case of gonorrhea will take hold, Dr. Miller says. Symptoms are more obvious in men than in women. Two to eight days after infection, a man will get a yellowish discharge from a reddened urethra and experience frequent, painful urination. Women's symptoms may include lower abdominal pain, a whitish vaginal discharge, abnormal uterine bleeding, and painful urination. But 10 to 30 percent of infected men and 70 to 90 percent of infected women don't have any symptoms.

Gonorrhea can spread and cause complications. Some infected women will develop pelvic inflammatory disease and inflammation of the fallopian tubes, which can cause ectopic pregnancy and permanent sterility. Sterility also can develop in men, and the infection can extend to the prostate and the rectum.

With such serious complications, treatment is essential. And the usual treatment is to nuke the gonococci with an enormous blast of penicillin. Why the A-bomb treatment?

The ingenious gonococci, it seems, have developed their own defense system. Their chromosomes have mutated so that antibiotics no longer can get inside the bacteria. Furthermore, many gonococci produce an enzyme to inactivate antibiotics that try to enter them.

So doctors now blast the disease with a minimum one-time dose of 4.8 *million* units of penicillin. The cure rate is better than 92 percent.

SYPHILIS

The syphilis bacteria, *Treponema pallidum,* is spreading like wildfire in the United States. Reported cases have doubled to more than 120,000 since 1985.

The first sign of syphilis is a painless sore, called a chancre, that appears usually three weeks after infection. In men, the sore is on or near the head of the penis. In women, it's usually on the labia, but it may be hidden inside the vagina. The sore heals in one to six weeks even without treatment. After a secondary stage in which lesions once again appear and heal without treatment, the disease enters a latency stage.

"In one-third of the people, the immune system – either macrophages or antibodies – wipes out the bacteria at this point," Dr. Miller says. "In the others, it kills most of the bacteria in the latency stage. But if there's no treatment, some bacteria survive and hide." When the bacteria come out of hiding and start multiplying, some people are at risk for the disease's tertiary symptoms, while others will go through life infected but without any damage.

Thankfully, syphilis isn't as smart as gonorrhea and is no match for antibiotics.

The number of people infected with syphilis has doubled since 1985.

CHLAMYDIA

The bacteria *Chlamydia trachomatis* cause the most common and one of the most damaging STDs in the United States. Three to four million Americans get chlamydia every year. It's the leading cause of pelvic inflammatory disease in women, and it can lead to male and female sterility.

Neutrophils gobble up chlamydia bacteria but don't kill them. Instead, the bacteria repro-

Chlamydia is the leading cause of pelvic inflammatory disease—a disease that leads to sterility.

duce inside the cells, killing them and releasing new bacteria. B-cells produce antibodies, but they're inadequate to the task.

Sixty-five percent of infected women have no symptoms; the others may have a fluid discharge. Men can have inflammation of the urethra and the epididymis, the long cord behind the testicles that transports sperm.

The treatment of choice is antibiotics – tetracycline, erythromycin, or doxycycline, taken orally. So far, the chlamydia bacteria show no resistance to these drugs. The cure rate is 95 percent.

PREVENTIVE ACTION

Either stick with one partner or make use of condoms, spermicides, and diaphragms, experts say.

The best way to avoid getting any STD is to not have sex. No sex, no transmission. However, this recommendation is not realistic, and certainly not necessary, for most people. Among those who are monogamous, there is no need to refrain from sex. The chances of getting an STD are slight. If you are not monogamous, experts recommend that you select your partners very carefully and that you make full use of condoms, spermicides, and diaphragms.

42

SLEEP:
REGENERATING
YOUR IMMUNE SYSTEM

It's 3:00 A.M. and you're snuggled into your pillow. You've cuddled up against your spouse, tucked the covers under your chin, and left your worries in another dimension. You're fast asleep, and nothing's going to move you until the alarm goes off at 7:00 A.M..

Your body is at rest – except for your immune system. It's not off duty with the rest of you. Not by a long shot. Even as you drift through those deep-sleep periods between dreams, your immune system is actually regenerating itself. It's taking all the proteins, fats, and carbohydrates you ate today and sending them to immunological fast-food restaurants throughout your body. And – freed of the competition from muscles and other systems that keep your body running throughout the day – your immune system is now gorging itself on the amino-acid McNuggets that are necessary to produce antibody warriors and their weapons.

When you're awake, every other part of your body gets to eat first. But when you're asleep, your immune system is first in the cafeteria line. Maybe that's why you get so sleepy when you're sick. Maybe your immune system needs an extra shot of O.J.

Your immune system does not go off duty when you sleep.

A NATURALLY OCCURRING
SLEEPING PILL

Maybe. And it may also be why your immune system has a way to put you to sleep – whether you like it or not – when it needs to regenerate.

How? "When you have an infection," explains Manfred L. Karnovsky, Ph.D., a biochemist at Harvard University, "the bacteria are attacked by your macrophages, which chew them up and release muramyl peptides, the building blocks of bacterial cell walls."

Your immune system even puts you to sleep when it needs to regenerate.

The peptides that escape the battlefield stimulate your immune system to produce more antibodies, then head for your brain and turn on your sleep switch. So not only does the peptide stimulate your immune system to build up its reserve troops, it also seems to assure you of a good night's sleep so the troops can get their rations.

In the long run, adds Dr. Karnovsky, muramyl peptides may even be able to be prescribed as a natural sleeping pill – a sleeping pill without the side effects or addictive potential of drugs now in use.

TEN WAYS TO SLEEP LIKE A BABY

Make sure you get the sleep you need to regenerate your healing forces.

But right now, cautions Dr. Karnovsky, "There are lots of enzymes between mouth and brain that can chop up the peptides." So until he and other researchers have figured out how to get the peptides where they're supposed to go, here's a ten-point plan to get the sleep that will allow your immune system to regenerate.

Avoid caffeine after dinner. Coffee, tea, cola, and other beverages that contain caffeine will zip you up for as long as 7 hours after you drink them.

Create a sleep sanctuary. Set aside your bed and bedroom for sleep and sex only. Don't watch TV, read, or work there.

Eat a bedtime snack. Don't eat a big meal before bedtime, but don't go to bed feeling hungry. The best kind of snack, doctors say, is a peanut butter sandwich or cheese and crackers topped off with a glass of milk.

Wake up at the same time every day. If you wake up at the same time every morning – even on weekends – you're more likely to get a good night's sleep. You'll also avoid the Monday morning "blahs."

Exercise. Regular exercise in the morning or late afternoon – never right before bed – can enhance sleep.

Know your sleep needs. Everybody requires a different amount of sleep. Sleep enough to feel alert and rested the next day – no more, no less.

Establish healthy sleep habits.

Keep your bedroom dark. Light is your body's cue that it's time to get up. Turn it off.

Avoid naps. Catnaps during the day or evening seem to fragment sleep at night. Avoiding them can keep you and your sleep together.

Make love, not war. Sleep after the deep release of an orgasm is practically automatic.

Develop a new bedtime ritual. An hour or so before bedtime, ease into a prebedtime ritual that will slide you into sleep. Play the same piece of music on a cassette deck, fold your mind into a relaxation mode, or journal away troublesome thoughts to a diary.

Then sleep the sleep of the innocent. It's the most regenerative of all.

43

SURGERY: STACKING THE DECK IN YOUR FAVOR

A typical operation gets under way.

A bright fall sun is flooding the two-story operating room, bouncing from tile to tile in the glistening white space until the entire room is filled with amplified light.

The nurse slaps a blood pressure cuff around your right arm, pumps it up until it strangles a blood vessel, then slowly lets out the air. Hssssssssss.

Another nurse picks up your left arm, expertly thumps the vein, then ties a tourniquet above your elbow. "Make a fist," she says as she thumps again. "That's it." You feel a needle prick. "Now release the fist."

Somewhere around your feet a nurse with a clipboard calls, "Name?" You tell her and carefully spell it out. "Operation?" A prickle of fear at your hairline. Doesn't she know?

You smile. Of course she does. It's just the hospital's way of double-checking. The blood pressure nurse moves away and the clipboard nurse moves up. She grasps your arm, carefully examines the patient information on your wristband and matches it to her charts. "Yep. That's you."

She moves away and another nurse takes her place, this one with a black rubber mask in one hand and a flexible hose in another. Now what?

290

The nurse patiently explains that she's going to hold the mask above your mouth and nose. She wants you to breathe deeply. You breathe. But with the second breath your lungs seem to hyperinflate. You can't get any air. You can't ask for help. And the operating room disappears into the deepest, darkest, blackest hole you've ever seen.

It's not like going to sleep.

The patient goes under.

A RISKY PROPOSITION

Every year more than 39 million people undergo surgery in the United States. And every year, the vast majority put their lives at unnecessary risk because of immune systems that are not up to the battle they're forced to fight.

The problem, explains Jack Jensen, M.D., a clinical professor of orthopedic surgery at the University of Texas Medical School, is that anesthesia, lack of sleep, stress, and poor nutrition – both before the surgery and in the hospital afterward – significantly increase your risk of complications and death by suppressing your immune system.

In an award-winning study conducted by Dr. Jensen and his colleagues at the University of Texas, for example, a preoperative assessment of 129 patients revealed that every single one of them was nutritionally depleted to some degree – even though their daily food intake averaged about 1,400 calories.

The majority of people undergoing surgery put themselves at risk because their immune systems are not ready for the fight.

RUNNING THE SURGICAL MARATHON

It's difficult to understand how someone eating almost 1,400 calories a day can be malnourished. But, as Dr. Jensen explains, anyone who is sick or injured generally has a metabolic need for between 2,000 and 2,400 calories – just about the same number that it takes to run a marathon.

The cellular warriors need nourishment.

What happens to your immune system when your body's running a deficit of 600 to 1,000 calories a day? Since the immune system is last in your body's chow line, it doesn't get fed. And when it doesn't get fed, it doesn't work. It slacks off. It makes fewer T-cell warriors. It decreases the amount of interferon messengers available. It forgets to tell the phagocytes how to kill. And all this just as a steel knife is about to slit your skin and allow a host of hospital-grown bacteria to breach the barricades.

Add to that the fact that major surgery itself has been shown to reduce your immune function by up to 50 percent. And factor in research reports that indicate that painkillers – like morphine – can reduce the function of individual immune players by 80 percent.

Total up these deficits, and you've got more than an unbalanced budget: You've got an immune system that, both before and after surgery, would have trouble fending off a wet dog, much less a platoon of deadly bacteria.

A PRE-OP CHECK

Ask your doctor for a pre-op check of immune function.

That's why anyone who's about to undergo surgery should ask their doctor to do a pre-op check of immune function, says Dr. Jensen. And that includes a skin test in which a substance that usually provokes your immune system to battle is scratched into your skin to see if your troops are on the alert. It also includes a blood test that will assess your nutritional state and actually count the number of immune system fighters – the white blood cells – in each drop of blood.

If either of these tests indicates you're not in tip-top condition, or if you've lost weight or been sick within the past 30 days or so, you should postpone the surgery until you've boosted your immune system back up to normal. "If your total lymphocyte count is less than 1,500 or if you had anergy [no response] to the skin tests," says Dr. Jensen, "you need to correct that before you get operated on. If you don't, statistically your chance of a complication is significantly higher."

Keep in mind that "complications" in the doctor business include life-threatening infections and death. In one study, for example, researchers reported that malnourished patients who underwent surgery with a low lymphocyte count were *20 times* more likely to die than patients without this risk factor. And another study, this one of 320 patients skin-tested before surgery at the University of Milan, revealed that the rate of sepsis – a serious blood infection that frequently kills older surgical patients – was almost *doubled* in those whose immune systems did not respond to the skin-test provocation.

TURNING YOUR IMMUNE POWER ON

Fortunately, there is a way to turn your immune power up to maximum just prior to your operation and stack the surgical deck in your favor. It's almost like preparing for a marathon. Only this time you're running for your life.

Load up on carbohydrates. Unless you're a diabetic, says Dr. Jensen, load your diet with carbohydrates the week before your surgery. That means lots of whole grains, fruits, and vegetables.

Unless you're diabetic, go for the carbohydrates.

Your body will store the carbohydrates as glycogen, then, when it needs an additional source of energy during and after surgery, it will burn the glycogen instead of protein. Then your body can use the postsurgical protein you eat for fighting off infections and repairing what your surgeon has sliced apart. The result? Possibly less time in the hospital.

This is no time to go on a diet.

Keep your calories between 2,000 and 2,400 a day. This is not the time to go on a diet, cautions Dr. Jensen. Your body needs every nutrient it can get. Post-op patients with poor pre-op nutrition spend nearly double the time in the hospital that well-nourished patients do – with double the complications.

When choosing what to eat, keep in mind that iron seems to be a particular concern. A study of 448 patients who underwent abdominal surgery at the University of Tampere, in Finland, for example, revealed that iron deficiencies increased hospital stays by an average of four days, increased the number of post-op infections by nearly 79 percent, and increased the number of deaths by 75 percent. The lack of iron depressed the patients' immune systems, concluded the researchers, and decreased the ability of the patients' blood to transport oxygen.

Take a multivitamin. Most people think they're eating three squares a day, says Dr. Jensen. They're not. Studies have shown that 20 percent of Americans, for example, eat their lunch at fast-food restaurants. Their chances of adequate nutrition, he believes, are slim. So cover your bases – and any possible deficencies – with a multivitamin.

Toast breakfast with a high-carbohydrate drink. Not *instead* of breakfast, mind you, but in addition. A high-carbohydrate breakfast drink helps keep your pre-op carbs and calories where they should be. And you don't need to ferret out a health food store to find a good one. The breakfast drinks right on your supermarket shelves – Carnation Instant Breakfast is the one he uses, says Dr. Jensen – are more than adequate.

Get your mind as ready as your body. The tension and worry surrounding any kind of surgery are enough to put several of your immune system players on the ropes. But the stresses of everyday life are the ones most likely to score an immune power knock-out.

Prime your mind.

In a study at the Veterans Administration Medical Center in Miami, for example, researchers found that men who were under a lot of life stress were likely to spend an extra five or six days in the hospital when they were operated on. They also had more complications and needed three times more painkillers than did men who were under less stress.

Stress robs your immune system of the power it needs.

That's why Dr. Jensen tries to get a sense of what's going on in the lives of his patients before he operates. And if a patient seems to be having a problem with his job, his wife, or something else in his life, Dr. Jensen will postpone the surgery and refer the patient to a clinical psychologist.

"Sometimes people are a little bit leery about going to a psychologist because they're not 'crazy,'" says Dr. Jensen. "But in the end, most people are really grateful, because the psychologists help them.

"When you get an 18-year-old kid who tears up his knee – he's a senior in high school and this is his big year – he's not gonna cry when he gets [to the surgeon] because he's a tough football player. He's okay, right?

"Baloney!" says Dr. Jensen. That boy's hurt. "He's not going to fulfill his dream in that part of his life – which is playing that senior year of football. So we're trying to get someone in there, someone the kid can talk to about what that injury means and how that changes his life."

Not only is that going to reduce the amount of stress the boy is experiencing and make a stronger patient, Dr. Jensen points out, it's also going to make a better person down the line. Because if that 18-year-old doesn't come to terms with not playing, "At age 30, at age 35, he's still trying to play that senior year. He's transferred it onto his kid who *has* to be the star football player because his dad never got to do it."

Patients who listened to taped healing messages during surgery got to go home faster.

Tune in a healing message. British patients who listened to taped healing messages – "You will not feel sick" or "You will not have any pain" – during surgery got to go home one to three days sooner than patients who had listened to blank tapes. The tuned-in patients actually healed faster. Why, scientists aren't sure. Could it be that their immune systems were listening?

Ask for a post-op roommate. A study of 27 men who underwent coronary bypass surgery in San Diego indicates that those who had a roommate who had already undergone surgery were less anxious before surgery, got out of bed faster after surgery, and went home sooner than bypass patients whose roommates had not had surgery yet. Whether these fast rebounders' immune power benefitted from less stress, or whether having a roommate who had already survived surgery gave them a sense of control over the outcome (which can also boost immune function), the researchers couldn't say. But the difference was so profound that they ended up recommending that all hospitals try to match "befores" with "afters."

Learn how to relax—and don't forget the tetanus shot.

Learn a relaxation technique. A study of 100 acutely ill patients at the University of Hawaii reveals that using a simple relaxation technique twice a day reduces the stressful effects of hospital noise by 34 percent. Since noise suppresses the immune system – and hospitals are full of beeps, burps, and buzzers – you might want to bone up on relaxation techniques like *Qigong* or Progressive Muscle Relaxation.

Check your tetanus protection. Although tetanus is rare, it has occurred following surgery, particularly surgery that involves the gastrointestinal tract. It's also hard to diagnose and is frequently fatal. Anyone undergoing abdominal surgery should consider getting a tetanus shot well before they hit the hospital, suggest researchers at the Mount Sinai School of Medicine in New York.

Be an optimist. A sense of optimism may block the immune-suppressive abilities of negative emotions, report researchers at the University of Miami and Carnegie-Mellon University. A study of 54 people who underwent heart surgery reveals that optimists healed faster, went home sooner, had fewer complications, and were significantly less likely to experience a heart attack after surgery than pessimists.

Optimists heal faster, go home sooner, and have fewer complications, one study showed.

Their strategy? "Prior to surgery," report the researchers, "optimists were much more likely to be making plans for themselves and setting goals for their recovery period than were pessimists." Pessimists tried to block out thoughts of what the recovery period might be like, while optimists were trying to gather as much information as possible.

Optimists knew they were going home. Pessimists were afraid they weren't.

ULCERS:
A POWERFUL NEW CURE

Bacteria may be responsible for many duodenal ulcers and for chronic gastritis.

"There's an old dictum in gastroenterology," says one researcher. " 'Once an ulcer, always an ulcer.' "

But new findings may chuck that dictum into a ditch. Because two Australian doctors have isolated a type of bacteria that they think may be responsible for many if not all duodenal ulcers and for chronic gastritis, a fancy term that means little more than inflammation of the stomach. Their theory is that standard treatment never eradicates the ulcer's *cause* (and maybe that's why 75 to 90 percent of all ulcers recur).

They also believe they've found a cure that is simple, inexpensive, and quick. It involves antibiotics and an over-the-counter medication that most of us have used at one time or another for upset stomach or traveler's diarrhea.

What is this common remedy? And what kind of bacteria trigger an ulcer? Let's take a look.

In 1979, when Robin Warren, a pathologist, and Barry Marshall, a gastroenterologist, were at the Royal Perth Hospital, Australia, they discovered that an odd strain of bacteria was present in nearly all the test samples from a group of patients with active chronic gastritis. Gastritis is a condition that frequently precedes or accompanies full-blown duodenal ulcer.

Over the next few years, Dr. Warren and Dr. Marshall tested hundreds of patients with gastritis and duodenal ulcer and found this spiral bacteria – which appeared to be a form of campylobacter – in most of them. The most common type of campylobacter bacteria is known to cause diarrhea in humans, so they named the new strain *Campylobacter pyloridis* because of its location in the stomach near the pylorus, the valve that holds food in the stomach.

A form of campylobacter was found in hundreds of patients.

They also began experimenting with a compound that had been shown to heal duodenal ulcer and, in fact, has a lower relapse rate than more conventional treatments. The substance is a compound of a heavy metal called bismuth, which had been used to treat syphilis and other bacterial infections before the discovery of penicillin in the 1940s. A very similar compound is the main ingredient of a common American over-the-counter remedy, Pepto-Bismol.

Patients responded well to a compound found in Pepto-Bismol.

What Dr. Marshall and Dr. Warren found was that, in a surprising number of cases, the bismuth compound worked. For many patients, not only did the bacteria disappear, but their ulcers did also. In fact, the researchers found that about 30 percent of ulcer patients who took the bismuth compound alone were clear of the bacteria, compared to none in the group given the usual ulcer treatment, cimetidine (Tagamet).

But the best clearance – 75 percent – came in the group given the bismuth compound and an antibacterial drug similar to a prescription medication sold in the United States under the trade name Flagyl.

Of course, the real test for any ulcer treatment is the relapse rate. "When we did the relapse study," reports Dr. Marshall, "we found the relapse rate was proportional to the number of patients who still had the germ after treatment.

Patients given the bismuth compound and an antibiotic fared better.

The relapse rate was between 80 and 100 percent in all the Tagamet patients. It was between 50 and 70 percent in the patients who got the bismuth and placebo. But the relapse rate was only about 30 percent in the patients who got the bismuth and antibiotic."

The Tagamet patients were subsequently given the antibiotic and bismuth, and, says Dr. Marshall, "they're all well. In fact, we have had hardly any patients requiring further treatment."

HOW IT WORKS

Campylobacter damages the lining of the stomach, leaving it open to irritation.

How does campylobacter cause gastritis and duodenal ulcer in the first place? Dr. Marshall and his colleagues believe the bacteria, which can live in the acid environment of the stomach, either digest or in some way damage the mucous lining of the stomach. Without that protective lining, which adheres to the stomach wall "like cling wrap," acid irritates and eventually eats a hole in the stomach, causing an ulcer.

The bacteria theory may explain why so many ulcers run in families. Scientists have long believed there was some genetic component to ulcers, though the exact connection has never been established. "We don't know how this bacterium is spread," says Dr. Marshall, "but there's some suggestion that it's through kissing, because husbands with duodenal ulcers often have wives who have gastritis. In fact, about half the wives of duodenal-ulcer patients have gastritis."

The cure is inexpensive.

One of the fortunate aspects of the Australian discovery – technically a rediscovery, since the bacterium was observed and promptly forgotten at least 40 years ago – is that the cure was not far behind. And it is an inexpensive cure. Conventional therapy, which includes indefinite maintenance, can cost roughly $1,000 or more over a period of 5 years, estimates Dr.

Marshall. "And even then you still get a high relapse rate," he says.

Campylobacter pyloridis is very suscepti-ble to the bismuth compound. Even if the anti-biotic stops working, as it sometimes does, the bismuth continues to fight the bacteria, says Dr. Marshall. The germs don't seem to build up any immunity to it. And bismuth is easily and inex-pensively available as Pepto-Bismol. "A two-week therapy of the bismuth compound and the antibiotic, which is really all that's usually needed, costs around $30," says the researcher. "And with this new therapy we're *curing* around 75 percent of the patients and the treatment doesn't have to go on for months.

"It's not just a treatment," emphasizes Dr. Marshall. "It's a cure."

Treatment with the bismuth/ antibiotic combination cures many patients.

45

VACCINES: HEDGING AGAINST INVASION

Vaccination is the superhero of the medical arsenal against disease. Its historical mission has been to protect the innocent and save lives. No red-caped comic book hero ever did a better job of it. Although it has been part of medicine's miraculous bag of tricks for almost 200 years, vaccination is ever new.

While today's scientists are busy formulating new vaccines for everything from tooth decay to genital herpes, they are also upgrading the old standbys. Wonderful vaccines that have turned the tide against some of humankind's most gruesome illnesses – polio, pertussis, cholera – are still haunted with the specter of rare, devastating side effects.

Scientists worldwide are laboring to make vaccines safer and more effective.

Scientists worldwide are laboring to make vaccines safer and more effective. Meanwhile, the average parent has more immediate concerns: Is it really safe to have my child vaccinated against pertussis? Should my elderly mother get those flu shots the doctor wants her to take every year?

It's more realistic to worry about the consequences of *not* being vaccinated, says one of the nation's top vaccine experts, John LaMontagne, Ph.D., director of the Microbiology and the Infectious Diseases Program of the National Institute of Allergy and Infectious Diseases. Before we give him his say, here's a refresher course on just why anyone would let a doctor needle them in the first place.

BAITING THE TRAIL

You get vaccinated for the same reason you let a bloodhound sniff an old sock. The canine nose needs only a whiff of the quarry in order to follow the bad guy's trail. When you get a vaccination, you are giving the soldier cells of your immune system a hint of what the enemy "smells" like.

A vaccination gives your immune system a look at the enemy.

Despite the bloodhound's awesome reputation for tracking, the dog has nothing over your immune system. Once alerted to a potential enemy, your immune system stays on the alert for years. In some cases, as in the vaccination for smallpox, cells that remember the enemy will circulate throughout your body on the lookout for smallpox virus for the rest of your life.

You think it's reaching to compare your immune system to a domestic animal? Guess again. Vaccination might be a fairly high-tech subject these days, but the word "vaccination" comes from the Latin word for "cow." You can't get any more domestic than that.

Almost 200 years ago, Edward Jenner created the first successful vaccine after noticing that milkmaids, who understandably spent a good deal of time in the company of cows, were immune to smallpox. Jenner surmised that exposure to the fairly innocuous cowpox somehow conferred immunity to the deadlier disease. He was right.

Today's vaccinations for a wide variety of diseases work for the same reasons that Jenner's smallpox inoculations worked in 18th-century England. Once your immune system responds to an infection, it remembers the substance that it had to deal with.

ON THE ROAD TO SAFETY

Your immune system receives a controlled dose of the infectious agent.

What vaccination does is give your immune system a controlled dose of the infectious agent. Once it comes in contact with a bit of dead or inactivated polio virus given in the form of a vaccine, for example, it is ever after on the lookout for polio virus.

That's the theory. And most of the time it works beautifully. But even so prestigious a publication as the *Journal of the American Medical Association* has published a study saying that: "Although currently available immunizing agents are both extremely safe and effective, they are neither completely safe nor completely effective."

Current vaccines are "neither completely safe nor completely effective," says one study.

Researchers are expecting that assessment to change soon.

"The science, perhaps I should say the art, of vaccine development is not perfect. It has grown enormously in the past few years," says Dr. LaMontagne.

An increased understanding of how the immune system works combined with new technology like genetic engineering is leading to a whole line of safer vaccines. Today's vaccines are safer than those of years past and the vaccines that should be available in the near future should be safer still.

The two vaccines that have generated the most concern among the general public in the past several years are pertussis vaccines for children and influenza vaccines.

KILLER WHOOPING COUGH

You don't hear much any more about pertussis, popularly known as whooping cough. That's a testimony to the success of the pertussis vaccine. You're more likely to hear an occasional horror story about severe reactions to the vaccine, including neurological complications, convulsions, uncontrolled screaming, and even a few deaths.

Reactions to the vaccine, although rare, are common enough that a few years back, vaccination rates fell off sharply in England, Japan, Denmark, and Sweden. People were afraid to have their children vaccinated. Pertussis epidemics soon followed.

Pertussis vaccines for children still generate controversy.

"Pertussis is a very serious infectious and epidemic disease," says Dr. LaMontagne. "Before this vaccine was developed, in the United States there were more than 200,000 cases a year and many, many deaths. Many people don't realize what a big problem it was not so long ago. The vaccine that is used in this country has had the profound effect of reducing our death rate from pertussis by almost 100 percent."

Physicians these days have a better understanding of when and how to administer the vaccine, says Dr. LaMontagne.

Before you have your child vaccinated with pertussis vaccine, discuss the possibility of adverse reactions to the vaccine with your pediatrician. The vaccine is administered in four separate doses given months apart. It is very important to mention any adverse reactions your child has to the vaccine to your doctor. In the event of a major reaction, he or she may decide against giving a second or third shot.

SIDESTEPPING INFLUENZA

Did the swine flu fiasco a few years back scare you out of taking your flu shots? The word from Dr. LaMontagne is: Not to worry. The cases of paralysis from Guillain-Barré syndrome that developed following the administration of that vaccine in 1976 were apparently limited to that particular vaccine.

Some cases of paralysis from Guillain-Barré syndrome followed the administration of flu vaccines in 1976.

"Why this occurred is still very much a mystery. Nobody really understands it. Influenza viruses, fortunately not the ones that affect man generally, do have a capacity to react with nervous tissue. It's not clear whether this might have been one of those phenomena. It is interesting to note that it occurred only in that year. There has not been any other association at any other time with any other influenza vaccine," says Dr. LaMontagne.

Current flu vaccines are considered very safe.

"Flu vaccines are very safe. I would say they are among the safest vaccines we use. Elderly people who do not get the flu vaccine are taking a very serious risk with their lives. Flu is a serious problem, and it can precipitate all kinds of other serious health problems that older people don't need to have. Everyone over the age of 65 should get a flu vaccine, as should people of any age who have an underlying chronic disease condition such as heart disease or cancer."

A new influenza vaccination is given every fall because the types of flu virus in the environment change every year. The flu bug is a little different each winter, so the vaccine to shoot it down has to be different, too.

SHOTS FOR CHILDREN

No matter what your personal feelings about vaccination, the fact remains that all states require proof of immunization before allowing a child to enter kindergarten or first grade. To find out about requirements in your state, contact your local public health department.

There is a problem with waiting until the child is about to enter school, however. The diseases that vaccinations protect against tend to be more severe in very young children.

A number of vaccinations are recommended for children.

The Centers for Disease Control recommends a standard schedule of vaccinations for children that will meet the requirements of most states.

DPT. This vaccine immunizes against diphtheria/pertussis/tetanus. It is administered at 2, 4, 6, and 15 months of age. Boosters of DPT should be given between the ages of 4 and 7. Boosters of diphtheria and tetanus should be administered again in ten years.

Polio. Immunization should be done at 2, 4, and 15 months. (If your infant receives the live polio vaccine, make sure that *all* members of the family have been immunized against polio. In a few isolated cases, the vaccine has caused polio in unprotected family members.) A booster shot should be given between the ages of 4 and 7.

MMR. This vaccine, for measles, mumps, and rubella, should be administered at 15 months.

Hib. This inoculation (*Haemophilus influenzaea* type b) should be administered at 18 months. It protects against the microbe that is a leading cause of meningitis in children.

SHOTS FOR ADULTS

"Adults hate to take shots. That's silly, particularly for something like polio, which is a more serious infection in adults than it is in children," says Dr. LaMontagne.

He recommends that all adults should make sure their immunizations are up to date for polio, tetanus, and diphtheria. He adds that women of childbearing age should be immunized against rubella, and people over 65 and high-risk people should be immunized for influenza and pneumococcal pneumonia.

One final note for travelers. Exotic places sometimes feature exotic microbes that can produce some very exotic diseases. Protect yourself by inquiring at your local public health department about recommended vaccinations well before you make your trip.

Adults must make sure their shots are up to date.

46

VIRUSES:
TROUBLE IN SMALL PACKAGES

Viruses don't have sex. And that's a big problem for all of us.

There are no such things as boy viruses or girl viruses. There are just viruses. And instead of being attracted to each other, they're attracted to you – to be more specific, to the cells of your immune system or your liver or your lungs or the membranes of your nasal passages.

Viruses *need* you in order to reproduce themselves.

Viruses *need* you in order to reproduce themselves. They can't do it alone.

"Bacteria reproduce by dividing themselves, one becomes two, two become four, and so on. Viruses actually go inside the body's cells. They take over all the machinery inside the cell to make new viruses. It's like an automobile assembly line," explains Byron Murray, Ph.D., professor of microbiology at Brigham Young University.

"Inside the cell, viruses make all the parts they need to reproduce themselves and then the parts come together. Viruses mature by assembly. So one virus can take over a cell and use it to produce thousands and thousands of viruses."

INVASION OF THE CELL SNATCHERS

Because viruses need you in order to carry on their own kind, they are always there, always seeking to get under your skin and slip into your very cells. What it all boils down to is that every day your immune system has to slug it out with an elusive enemy much smaller than yourself. Most of the time you win, fortunately. But no sooner is the battle finished than villainous viruses are at their mischief again.

Did we say *small?*

Viruses are anywhere from 10 to 1,000 times smaller than bacteria. And bacteria are microscopic, single-celled animals. The polio virus, one of smallest of the small, is so tiny that if you picture an *E. coli* bacterium to be the size of a football field, then the virus would be about the size of a football. (*E. coli* bacteria live by the millions in your intestines.)

It's no wonder this enemy is so elusive and that medical weapons to help the body fight back are so difficult to come by. Although viruses have been on the attack for millennia, it was only at the turn of the century that they were discovered. And it's a relatively recent development that allowed scientists to get their first look at them.

When scientists first trained their electron microscopes on viruses, they saw something that doesn't even look alive. Some viruses look like tiny faceted gemstones, others like shuttle craft from some futuristic starship. The AIDS virus looks like a miniature sputnik, the rabies virus like a bullet. They aren't even single-celled organisms, just a bit of genetic information wrapped up in a protein coat.

"They're strange. A lot of people don't consider viruses to be living entities. I personally do," says Dr. Murray.

THE DEADLIEST EMBRACE

Because of the – you'll pardon the expression – intimate relationship that viruses have with

Viruses are anywhere from 10 to 1,000 times smaller than bacteria.

A lot of people don't consider viruses to be living entities.

you, they are particularly difficult to deal with.

There is not much in a virus that can be attacked with drugs. Viruses use the chemistry and machinery of your own cells, so drugs that attack them tend to be toxic to human cells as well.

"It's not difficult to find a compound that will inhibit the virus. That's extremely easy. It's very difficult to find one that will inhibit the virus and not damage the cell. That's why there's just a handful of antiviral drugs around today," explains Dr. Murray.

A drug like acyclovir, which is used for herpes, is relatively nontoxic. But something like AZT, used to treat AIDS, is toxic and plagued with side effects, says Dr. Murray.

"Without AIDS, we wouldn't be using AZT. When a disease is life-threatening, you have to look at the risk/benefit ratio," he says. "AZT has considerable side effects, but if you're going to die of AIDS, it's better to prolong life than to die. You wouldn't use AZT for herpes fever blisters."

Dr. Murray expects a number of antiviral drugs to be developed in the near future, many of them as "spin-off compounds" from AIDS research.

In the meantime, treating viral infections comes down to the same regimen that doctors have prescribed for years: getting plenty of rest and good nutrition while letting nature take its course. Drugs currently given during viral infections are to relieve the *symptoms* of the disease; they don't go after the viruses themselves in the same way that antibiotics mop up bacteria.

When viruses come knocking at your door and end up in an intimate embrace with your body's cells, you can't yet reach into your medicine cabinet for quick relief. Someday you may be able to send those unwanted intruders packing. Until then, "Take two aspirins and . . ."

There is not much in a virus that can be attacked with drugs.

Treating a virus involves getting plenty of rest and good nutrition while letting nature take its course.

47

WARTS: AN AMAZING DISAPPEARING ACT

Touch a toad and you might get one. But then again, if you already have one and you rub it with the skin of a chicken gizzard and hide the skin under a rock, it might go away.

The subject is warts, of course, the unsightly growths famous for perching on witches' noses and otherwise tormenting just plain folks. Just plain folks have been dealing with them for centuries and have come up with more folksy cures than you can shake a stick at. (Speaking of shaking sticks, it's said that if you cut one notch in a persimmon-wood stick for every wart that you have, those warts should clear right up.)

So what's this weird stuff about warts doing in a book about the immune system?

It seems a lot of those oddball folk cures sometimes work, and they work in ways that might teach us a lot more about manipulating our immune defenses.

For years, medical science has tried to explain away these cures by pointing out that warts have a high rate of spontaneous remission. The cure becomes a nice, comfortable "coincidence." And that makes it okay for doctors to tell their own favorite wart-cure stories and to share a laugh.

A few researchers aren't laughing anymore. They've studied the effects of hypnosis and suggestion, and they've found that warts frequently *do* respond.

There are a lot of folk cures for warts—and many of them work.

WHISKING AWAY WARTS

Folk cures for warts should be the subject of serious scientific study to find out *why* and *how* they work, says Andrew Weil, M.D., author of *Health and Healing,* a book that examines alternative healing practices. Dr. Weil, who is associate professor of the Division of Social Perspective in Medicine at the University of Arizona, maintains that studying wart cures could yield vitally important information to medical science.

Some researchers are beginning to study why folk cures work.

Here we have warts, contagious growths that are associated with a family of viruses known as human papilloma virus (HPV). When any wart is examined, it's shown to be infected with HPV. Very real. Very material. Yet warts have been cured by such bizarre behavior as rubbing them with a potato and burying the potato under the right kind of tree at a certain phase of the moon, says Dr. Weil.

These cures must involve the mind/body connection.

How and why such peculiar treatments work is not known, but the cure must involve the mind/body connection – the tie-ins between the brain, nervous system, circulatory system, and immune system, says Dr. Weil.

Unlike spontaneous cures of cancer – which are rare but do happen – spontaneous cures of warts are common enough that they could be produced repeatedly in a laboratory setting, maintains Dr. Weil. That would enable researchers to study the mechanics of such cures, including temperature changes, immune system changes, and a whole gamut of possible variables.

"It's especially silly that we don't pay a lot of attention to this," says Dr. Weil.

THE MEDICAL CHALLENGE

Meanwhile, medical science is not doing particularly well with its own set of scientific wart cures. Physicians attack warts in a variety of ways, trying everything from slicing them away to zapping them with lasers.

Yet currently available treatments tend to be painful and only partially effective. Scarring is a problem. And there are frequent recurrences. Warts are hard to get rid of and tend to come back after treatment.

Currently available medical treatments tend to be painful and only partially effective.

Before you take your warts to a physician, suggests Dr. Weil, go ahead and try a folk cure. Ask around among your friends and family until you find a cure that you can get emotionally involved with. It should either appeal to you, scare you, or disgust you. The emotional involvement seems to be the key, says Dr. Weil. If one cure doesn't work, try a couple more, he says. It can't hurt you, and it just might work.

So when the moon is full and the frost is on the pumpkin, find a big white rock next to a crossroads and . . . Sorry, but you're supposed to find your own cure.

48

YEAST INFECTIONS: RISING TO THE CHALLENGE

Many women are desperate for relief from yeast infections.

Dateline, Utah. Summer of 1988. A suburban housewife accidentally sets her kitchen on fire trying to rid her life of yeast infections once and for all.

You think yeast infections are embarrassing?

Try explaining to a group of firemen that the reason you put your panties in the microwave in the first place was because a University of Florida study proved that microwaving freshly laundered cotton panties on high for 5 minutes kills yeast. You *thought* the panties were cotton; how were you supposed to know they were going to burst into flames and set your kitchen on fire?

Our intention in resurrecting this story – one that this Utah housewife probably wishes would die – is not to snicker at her error, amusing though it is in retrospect. It just serves to show that women are desperate for relief. Women are so desperate that they will try anything and buy anything that promises relief from the itching and burning misery of vaginal yeast infections.

And these days there are a lot of people out there promising relief and selling remedies. Popular advice books turn fighting the yeast beast into a lifestyle. Cookbooks for eliminating yeast (and we don't mean just from bread) offer extensive menu-planning assistance. Antiyeast nutrients, lotions, and potions compete for space in specialty shops.

If women are confused about yeast, it's not surprising, says Marjorie Crandall, Ph.D. Many physicians are also confused by conflicting and sometimes controversial claims. For while yeast infection is prevalent, misinformation about yeast infection is downright rampant, she warns. Dr. Crandall, who knows the agony of recurrent yeast infections from firsthand experience, is a woman whose extensive research on yeast has led her to leave Harbor-UCLA Medical Center to set up her own Yeast Consulting Services in Torrance, California. She is also working on a book about yeast infections.

There is a lot of confusion about the causes of and treatments for yeast infections.

FUNGUS RUNS RAMPANT AMONG US

While physicians are still slugging it out over the yeast syndrome controversy – about which symptoms can be attributed to yeast and whether special diets help – there is one thing they all seem to agree on: Yeast infections are a problem for a whole lot of women. A big problem.

Yeast infections are extremely common.

Most of the time, when a person has a yeast infection, the culprit is a fungus known as *Candida albicans.* Candidal infections are more common than all other fungal infections combined. And vaginal candidiasis is one of the most frequently diagnosed diseases in gynecology. Three out of four women will experience this infection at least once during their childbearing years. And at any given time, 6 percent of all women of childbearing age are suffering from the infection.

Nor is the yeast problem limited to women. Both men and women can suffer from intestinal yeast overgrowth, says Dr. Crandall. And men can get a genital form of yeast infection. Although there are frequently no symptoms, a man can pass the yeast back to his sexual partner. A woman whose candidal infection is successfully treated can be reinfected this way again and again.

Men can have an infection without experiencing any symptoms.

"I call it sexual Ping-Pong," says Dr. Crandall. "Yet yeast infection is not treated as a sexually transmitted disease. Physicians usually don't treat the man, which is unfortunate."

Speaking of sexually transmitted disease, it is not uncommon these days for women to respond to a yeast infection diagnosis with sheer panic, says Dr. Crandall. Many have read that yeast infection is often the first sign of AIDS in women. Don't panic. Yeast might be the first thing that women with AIDS get, but it doesn't follow that if you have yeast vaginitis, AIDS must be around the corner.

HOW TO TELL IF IT'S YEAST

Yeast infection symptoms range from itching to pain during sexual intercourse.

The main symptoms of vaginitis caused by yeast infection are itching, discharge, inflammation, and swelling, says Dr. Crandall. Also possible are a burning sensation during urination, pain during sexual intercourse, a white vaginal discharge that resembles cottage cheese, and sometimes a yeasty, breadlike odor. A man with a genital yeast infection might experience a burning sensation during ejaculation, if he feels anything at all.

If the yeast infection is in the intestines, both men and women might experience any combination of these symptoms: acid stomach, indigestion, abdominal pain, constipation (more often), diarrhea (less often), anal itching, and occasionally even symptoms of drunkenness.

Many things besides yeast cause vaginitis.

But take note. There are all kinds of things that might cause vaginitis besides yeast. And there are all kinds of health problems that can produce the indigestion-type symptoms described above.

So how do you know it's yeast?

Ah, you don't. You just can't diagnose a yeast infection by symptoms alone, or with the help of books, magazine articles, and well-meaning advice from your friends.

"People cannot diagnose themselves," warns Dr. Crandall. "That's the problem with this yeast syndrome business. People read all these books and they think, 'I have candida,' and then they go to their friendly nutritionist and they get all kinds of nutritional supplements and spend a lot of money on those. They could really jeopardize their health, especially because they might not have candida at all. They may have some other problem that might be more serious."

So, rule number one in dealing with *Candida albicans* is: Don't make any assumptions. Dr. Crandall recommends that you take your suspicions to your family physician who is familiar with your complete medical history. Your family doctor will know about things that might predispose you to yeast infection, such as past use of antibiotics, cortisone, or birth control pills.

Only health professionals can diagnose yeast infection.

"Recurrent vaginal candidiasis or chronic intestinal candidiasis is both an infection by candida and an allergy to candida. So you have to treat both, and that can be a problem," says Dr. Crandall. "If you go to a family doctor, she or he is trained just to treat the infection. My contribution in this field is to point out to patients and physicians alike that this is also an allergy to the infective agent. So you have to treat the allergy component as well as treating the infection."

Diagnosing candida infection is not always easy, Dr. Crandall maintains. All of us have some candida in us. It is just one of those ever-present microbes with which we share our environment. A woman not suffering candidiasis symptoms might easily test positive for candida. At the same time, a person who is allergic to candida might suffer the full-blown range of symptoms with very little yeast actually present to account for it. In the past, such patients might have been sent to a psychologist. A more appropriate referral might be to an allergy specialist, maintains Dr. Crandall. Once candida allergy or allergy to

Sometimes it takes specialists to make a proper diagnosis.

other yeasts and molds is diagnosed, a person can be desensitized to the substances.

FIGHTING THE YEAST BEAST

If you are plagued by recurring yeast infections, don't lose hope. Besides cooperating with your physician in your antiyeast treatment, there are all kinds of ways that you can fight back.

Dr. Crandall has put together an exhaustive list of do's and don'ts.

Don't use chemical irritants on the genital area.

Avoid chemical irritants. Don't use any over-the-counter vaginal products, including douches, creams, jellies, deodorants, or sprays. Don't swim in chlorinated swimming pools or soak in hot tubs or spas. Don't use perfumed or colored toilet paper. Presoak and hand-scrub your panties, then wash them with unscented detergent (don't use fabric softener), and be sure to rinse well. Don't use bath oils, shampoos, or soaps on the genital area.

"My recommendation is, don't use anything at all to wash except water," says Dr. Crandall. "Women have bought into this concept that they have to use soap and deodorant and perfumes and all these things to make that part of their body smell like strawberries or roses or whatever, and that's not natural. It's not healthy.

"The bacteria in your vagina keep you healthy by preventing the overgrowth of not just yeast but other pathogens as well. My rule of thumb is, don't put anything in your vagina you wouldn't put in your eye."

Keep cool and dry. Wear only nonrestrictive, white cotton underwear. Don't wear tight jeans and don't wear panty hose under slacks. Make sure that panty hose have a cotton crotch.

Practice safe sex and watch your diet.

Practice safe sex. Ask your sex partner to use a condom. Wash before as well as after sex. Void your bladder both before and after intercourse. Avoid sex if you have vaginitis.

Avoid yeasts in foods. "Certain foods and airborne allergens will cause allergic reactions in women who have recurrent vaginal yeast infections and in men and women who have chronic intestinal candidiasis," says Dr. Crandall. "So don't eat any foods containing yeasts or molds, including bread, doughnuts, beer, wine, vinegar, pickles and other fermented foods, cheeses, mushrooms, yeast extract, fruits with molds on their surfaces, and fruit and vegetable juices."

Avoid excessive sweets. Although still controversial, there is research showing that *excessive* sweets can contribute to ycast infections in susceptible women, says Dr. Crandall.

Use antibiotics correctly. Improper use of antibiotics can lead to yeast infections.

ADDITIONAL HELP IS ON THE WAY

Research continues into the possible causes and cures for recurrent yeast infections, with some researchers looking at the connections between yeast infections and the immune system.

One Cornell University study notes that yeast infections are associated with immune system suppression. Modulating immune system functioning with such agents as ibuprofen (such as Advil) may prove to be helpful treatment in conjunction with antifungal medication, the study suggests.

Other studies have noted zinc deficiency problems in women with recurrent candidiasis. Zinc deficiency "may be a contributing factor," one study notes.

While the answers to the causes and cures of yeast infections are still rolling in, there is already a whole lot you can do. You don't need to give in to the yeast beast. Fight back.

Yeast infections are associated with immune system suppression, one study notes.

Part III
How to Build a Strong Immune System

49

YOUR 30-DAY IMMUNE POWER PROGRAM

You've learned about vaccines, protective veggies, smoke-free environments, and regular checkups. You've discovered the regenerative magic of positive feelings, relaxation, and sound sleep. You've even come to realize how everyday stress can knock your immune system's defensive players to the ground – and how a simple laugh can help bounce them back into action.

But how do you take all the bits and pieces of this immune power puzzle and put them together? How do you actually build a strong immune system?

Now that you know about the immune system, you want to know how to make it stronger.

By following this 30-day immune power program. Using the nine most important ideas suggested by the doctors, scientists, and researchers interviewed for this book, the 30-day program provides step-by-step, one-day-at-a-time instruction to help you build a stronger immune system. Here's the lineup for what are called the nine immune power principles.

THE NINE IMMUNE POWER PRINCIPLES

1. Develop the power of positive feeling.
2. Feed your T-cells top-level nutrition.
3. Take a vacation from stress.
4. Program your immune system for optimum power.

There are nine principles to employ.

5. Set up an exercise program you'll stick to.
6. Regenerate your immune system with sleep.
7. Use preventive medicine to give your body a fighting chance.
8. Take control of your personal environment.
9. Reach out to the folks around you.

Following this guide will set your immune system for maximum power.

How do you implement these power principles? Follow the day-by-day guide on the following pages and chart your progress with the quizzes at the end of each 7-day period. In 30 days, you should have an immune system better able to do what it was designed to do: resist everything from marauding microbes to prowling protozoa. In 30 days, your immune system will be set for maximum power.

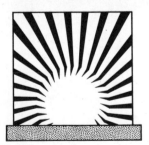

DAY 1   Start a Journal

What does a journal have to do with setting your immune power on max? That's what James W. Pennebaker, Ph.D., keeps asking himself – and every student he can draft into studies at Southern Methodist University in Dallas, where he's a professor of psychology.

His first study, Dr. Pennebaker says, found that writing about painful personal problems – and the way you feel about them – can actually bolster your immune system. In that first study, 25 students were asked to write out their feelings about problem situations that they hadn't been able to resolve, spending 20 minutes a day for four days at the task. Another group of 25 students wrote for the same time period but wrote about unimportant topics.

Blood samples taken just before and just after the experiment, as well as six weeks later, showed that students who wrote out their negative feelings had an increased T-cell response. Those who recorded thoughts on trivial subjects showed no such improvement. Six weeks later, the "confiding" students still had stronger immune defenses.

Students who wrote about negative feelings had an increased T-cell response.

A hyped-up immune response should translate into a healthier student. But to make sure, Dr. Pennebaker divided 130 incoming freshman into two groups and verified the results of his study.

"People think that everybody loves college," chuckles Dr. Pennebaker, "but that's a lie." It's a very stressful time. And since stress is known to suppress the immune system, what better way to see if recording a history of that difficult time can offset the effects of stress and zip up the immune system?

In this second study, Dr. Pennebaker asked one of the student groups to write out their feelings about school for 20 minutes a day over a three-day period. Individuals in the second group were told to write only about inconsequential matters and not deal with their feelings at all. Each group began the three-day period at different times during the semester.

In one study, students wrote about the stresses of starting college.

After the study, Dr. Pennebaker checked with the University health service and compared the number of "sick calls" students in each group had made to the infirmary. The results? Students who documented their stress about coming to college had significantly fewer health problems, and remained healthier up to five months later, than those who had written of trivial things.

Students who kept journals had significantly fewer health problems.

Apparently writing about a stressful event immediately after it happens does counteract the suppressive effects of stress on your immune system.

CATCH A SCREAM
BETWEEN THE PAGES

How can you use a journal to enhance *your* immune response? As diarist Tristine Rainer suggests in her book *The New Diary:* "Instead of screaming or going to the window and shooting a gun wildly into the street, I put the scream in the diary, catch it between the pages, close the book tight, and go on."

Pour your emotions out on paper every day.

Easier said than done, right? But as another experienced diarist suggests, "Go through the motions and you'll get the emotions." And the motions are not that difficult. Some people who keep journals say that it's helpful to go to the same quiet "writing spot" every day, set the writing mood by putting on an instrumental tape or record, and then write your heart out for the next 15 minutes.

Or just write when something really gets you down.

The end of the day is a natural time for some to look back and sort out their feelings. Others find that, because of work or family responsibilities, keeping a journal is easier if they integrate it *into* their day. A secretary, for example, might write on her lunch hour. A mother might write during baby's naptime. Or a police officer might write after he or she hands in the daily report. In any case, you don't have to write every day to get the health benefits of keeping a journal, says Dr. Pennebaker – just when something bothers you or gets you down.

Keeping a journal is a process of self-discovery.

But don't be surprised if you find yourself *wanting* to write every day. Documenting the events in your life and the way you feel about them is a process of self-discovery, and that can be exciting. As one diarist observes: "Making entries in a journal is like digging a garden. Just turning the soil may reveal a treasure that lies close to the surface."

Learn an Active Relaxation Technique

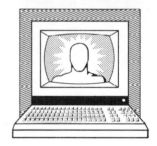

DAY 2

The first breath of light touches the high-peaked roofs of Beijing, shimmers down the gray walls of the city's courtyards, and pauses in the branches of a thousand willow trees planted along the river. The river – actually a wide moat that encloses the ancient palaces of China's emperors – changes from black to slate to gray as the light begins to penetrate its surface.

It's early, and most of the city is still asleep. But under the graceful willows of Beijing, equally graceful movements reveal a quiet army of dark-eyed people clad in baggy pants, oversized jackets, and canvas shoes.

Some move smoothly in ancient patterns of physical harmony, others stand still as statues. But whether there is movement involved or not, each is performing *Qigong,* the traditional deep-breathing exercises that create the kind of total relaxation that underlies a unified state of mental and physical harmony.

It is this kind of relaxation, scientists say, that keeps your immune system on its toes. And the Chinese have been masters of it for centuries.

Chinese people exercise at dawn.

They are performing *Qigong,* a relaxing breathing exercise that can help the immune system.

Try a relaxing American version of *Qigong*.

To try an Americanized version of *Qigong*, stretch out on your bed or floor, with your legs extended, arms at your sides, and your head resting on a pillow. Then close your eyes and slightly clench your teeth. The tip of your tongue should touch the hard palate, just behind your upper front teeth.

Breathe normally through your nose, slowly and evenly. Now focus on the word "calm" as you inhale. Focus on the word "relax" as you exhale. Then silently instruct each part of your body to relax. Say to yourself, "Head – relax." "Neck – relax." "Shoulders – relax." "Arms – relax."

Continue all the way down your body to your toes, then repeat the entire exercise. It should be done once or twice a day for 30 minutes at a time, working up to a maximum of three or four times a day, 20 to 30 minutes at a time.

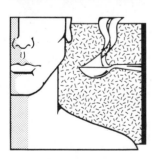

DAY 3

Put the B Vitamins to Work

Breakfast at Flo's. Lunch by the vending machine. Dinner courtesy of a microwavable cardboard container. How's your immune system supposed to keep up its strength?

The problem is that it's always last in your body's chow line when the nutrients are passed out. So if you don't eat enough – or enough of the right foods – your immune system's going to think you've given it a furlough. Then when a viral or bacterial invader decides to test your defenses, some of your antibody warriors will still be in the barracks – too weak to launch an attack.

One way to put some starch in your warriors is to put some starch in your diet. And that means the right kinds of starch: whole grain breads, pastas, and cereals – with a little wheat germ thrown in for good measure. The key ingredients here are the B vitamins, which are also found in beef and dairy products.

Your immune system requires B vitamins.

Fortunately, other good sources of B vitamins are also easy to integrate into your life: Chick-peas tossed in your salad, sunflower seed snacks on your coffee table, navy bean soup on a cold day, or a salmon steak grilled outside on a hot one – all combine to keep your immune system on the alert. You might also want to dine on chicken breast or beef liver occasionally, since they're particularly good souces of vitamin B_6 – a nutrient your immune system just can't do without.

How much of the B vitamins do you need? A safe bet is to follow the U.S. Recommended Daily Allowance (USRDA) established by the Food and Drug Administration. The USRDA for B_2, for example, is 2 milligrams daily – about the same amount found in either 14 ounces of chicken breast meat or 7 or 8 ounces of cooked beef liver.

Fourteen ounces of anything is a little hard to swallow, of course – which is why you should choose the sources of your B vitamins carefully. You need so much food just to get your body's recommended allowances that you'll end up feeling like a stuffed turkey if you don't make an effort to get the most vitamin for the least food.

Learn the foods that provide you with optimum amounts of B vitamins.

So think carefully about what you eat. Some examples of food sources and serving sizes that provide the USRDA's for the rest of the B's are listed in the table below.

Vitamin	USRDA	Source
Thiamine (B_1)	1.5 mg	1 tbsp. brewer's yeast ½ cup dried sunflower seeds 1 cup Product 19 cereal 1 cup Total cereal
Riboflavin (B_2)	1.7 mg	1½ oz. cooked beef kidneys 1½ oz. cooked beef liver
Niacin	20 mg	7 oz. roasted chicken breast 1 cup dry-roasted peanuts 12 oz. canned white tuna (water-packed)
Folate	400 mcg	½ cup simmered chicken livers 4 tsp. brewer's yeast 1½ cups boiled spinach
B_{12}	6 mcg	⅓ oz. cooked beef liver 4 oz. sockeye salmon 1 or 2 steamed clams 1½ cups cooked lobster 3 oz. steamed crabmeat 8 oz. cooked pot roast
Pantothenate	10 mg	1½ cups simmered chicken livers 1½ cups cooked wild rice

Sound like a lot of food? Now you know why scientists say your body's nutritional needs are such that you can't afford to eat junk. You simply can't afford the "empty" calories. And remember – it's your immune system that gets fed last.

Develop an Image of Health

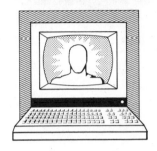

DAY 4

Now that you know how to put your body into a state of deep relaxation, you're ready to tell your immune system exactly what you expect it to do. You're ready to tell it to mobilize its forces, reconnoiter the territory, and target the enemy. But how can you talk to a bunch of T-cells?

Scientists tell us that by using imagery – forming a series of mental pictures that translate your words into patterns your body can understand – you can order your immune system up to optimum power. Think of it as programming a computer and you've got the general idea. The only difference is that instead of using the computer's mathematical languages, you'll use your body's language of images.

But your conversation with your body doesn't begin with "Hello." It begins with a relaxation exercise. So put yourself into the deeply relaxed mode that you learned on Day 2 of this program. Then either focus on the image beginning on page 178 or develop one of your own. If you make up your own, however, remember that the key to revving up your T-cells is to visualize them working to keep you healthy and then see yourself as having achieved that state – even if you presently have a chronic illness.

A middle-aged woman with rheumatoid arthritis in her wrists and knees, for example, worked with Gerald N. Epstein, M.D., an assistant clinical professor of psychiatry at Mount Sinai Medical Center in New York, to develop an

You communicate with your immune system through images.

image that would shrink an 8-inch rheumatoid nodule in her right knee.

In her visualization, which Dr. Epstein reported in the journal *Advances,** the woman lay on her back at the beach right at the point where sand and water flowed in and out of one another in a constant dance of give and take. The sky was a cloudless blue, the sun was bright and gold, and pointing her toes toward the water, the woman covered herself with wet sand, leaving only the soles of her feet and her head exposed to the sun.

A woman with rheumatoid arthritis used an image of herself lying in the sun.

Then, as she watched, the tide came in and entered imaginary holes in the soles of her feet. She sensed spiral currents of water as they washed the inside of her feet, dissolving any deposits, eliminating toxins, and clearing away any accumulations. Then as the tide began to go out, the water slowly flowed back out of the woman's feet – taking with it accumulated debris that was now nothing more than gray or black streaks being carried away on the outgoing tide.

The woman watched as the tide came in and entered her feet a second time, this time rising as high as her ankles. It retreated, then came in a third time, going all the way up to her knees, where the spiral currents of water massaged the muscles, stretched the ligaments, and cleaned the cartilage and kneecaps until they were gleaming white.

She visualized the tide coming in and soothing her knees.

When the tide retreated once again, the woman felt the spiral currents reversing, slowly flowing back down through her legs and calves, into her ankles, her feet, and out through the holes in her soles. Once again she saw the wastes

She imagined the rheumatoid nodules leaving her with the receding tide.

*Adapted and used with permission from "The Image in Medicine: Notes of a Clinician," by Gerald N. Epstein, M.D., *Advances,* vol. 3, no. 1, Winter 1986. Copyright 1986, Institute for the Advancement of Health.

emerge as black or gray streaks being carried away on the outgoing tide. But this time, as Dr. Epstein suggested, she imagined that all the rheumatoid nodules went with the tide.

Once the nodules disappeared, the woman stood up, dived into the ocean, and swam to the horizon, visualizing her arms, legs, and torso as being immensely long and fluid. When she reached the horizon, she flipped over on her back and returned to shore using the backstroke. She emerged from the water, paused to let the sun dry her off, then donned a robe left on the sand. Finally, she sat down, exhaled, and opened her eyes.

The woman used this imagery three times a day for three months, Dr. Epstein reports, then returned to her rheumatologist for an evaluation. The result? The nodule in her right knee had shrunk by almost 3½ inches.

Her body had understood the image.

With repeated use of the image, the nodule in her right knee shrank.

Supercharge Your Sex Life

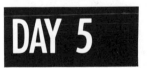

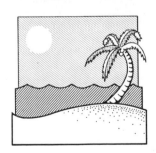

When used to intensely communicate love and caring from one human being to another, sex may trigger chemical changes in your body that can actually enhance your immune system, says Detroit psychologist Paul Pearsall, Ph.D. It apparently keeps your hormones – which we now know directly affect the immune system – in a "just right" balance that helps fight the negative effects of stress on a chemical level.

How can you take advantage of this built-in immune booster? The first step is to take responsibility for your own sexuality, suggests Dr. Pearsall in his book *Superimmunity.* "Express your needs directly and openly and communicate freely about contraception, disease, responsibility, religious conviction, and expectations between yourself and your partner."

To improve your sex life, learn to communicate.

Easier said than done, of course. But, "the bottom line in developing a more satisfying sexual relationship is a couple's ability to talk with each other," says Wallace Denton, Ed.D., professor and chairman of the Department of Family Therapy at Purdue University. Unfortunately, "People seem to be able to talk about sex in animals and sex in other people, but when it comes down to talking about 'you and me, Honey,' that's another story."

So here are six suggestions to get the talk flowing.

Choose the right moment to let your partner know what you are saying is important.

Pick the right time. "We sometimes can shoot ourselves down by simply approaching a person at the wrong time," says Dr. Denton. "A husband, for example, who wants to talk with his wife about their sexual relationship while she's preparing the evening meal is a natural-born loser. She's got six things on her mind at that moment, and not one of them is her sex life."

Make it very clear that you're talking about something important. "A lot of times people start talking with their mate about something that's important to them, but the other one doesn't recognize that this is something that's really important," says Dr. Denton. "You can't communicate until you've got the other person's attention. So you say something like, 'Honey, when you have time I've got something really important that I'd like to talk about.'"

Defuse the situation. "If you're pretty sure the other person's going to be angry or get upset," says Dr. Denton, "You can say, 'This is something we've talked about before. I hope you won't get angry. I really would like for you to listen to me and when I get through talking, I'll listen to you.' "

Don't be negative. "Instead of saying, 'I think we need to improve our sex life,' put it on a positive note," says Shirley Zussman, Ed.D., a sex and marital therapist in New York City and codirector of the Association for Male Sexual Dysfunction. Say, "There are a lot of things that are enjoyable about our sex life, and I'd like to open up some ways in which we can make it even better."

Make your approach positive.

Don't talk away your time. "If you've talked more than about 2 or 3 minutes, then you've probably talked too long," Dr. Denton says. "Sometimes we need to stop and let the other person talk."

Share a good book. If you and your mate still have trouble talking about sex, try reading a book or article on the subject together. "That's one step removed and might allow a couple to share different opinions about what they're reading," says Raul Schiavi, M.D., professor of psychiatry and director of the Human Sexuality Program at Mount Sinai School of Medicine in New York. "That might facilitate talk about themselves."

If you really can't talk, try reading a book or article on the subject together.

Sneak Exercise into Your Life

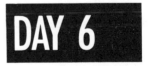

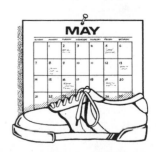

Buy a dog. Sell your car. Move into a five-story condo. Do whatever it takes to get your feet moving, and your immune system will thank you. That's because moderate amounts of exercise do more than move your feet. They also keep your immune system in motion by speeding the flow of blood throughout your body. And that can shorten the response time of antibodies as they zip around with it.

Moderate amounts of exercise also seem to stimulate your body's production of beta endorphins, substances that – in labs at the National Institutes of Health, at least – latch onto natural killer cells and increase their ability to destroy invaders by an average of 63 percent.

But who's got time for exercise? Nobody. So here are some ways to sneak it into your life.

Walk with your friends and walk on your errands.

Turn your phone friends into walk friends. Instead of picking up the phone to yak with a friend during an afternoon break, follow the phone company's advice to "reach out and touch someone" more explicitly: Ask the friend to meet you on a corner and go for a walk. You'll be reenergized by both the walk and the company.

Walk your errands. Whether you do errands on your lunch hour, on weekends, or on your way home from work, consider walking your errands rather than "running" them in the car. If you prefer to pick up several items in a mall or shopping center, choose a distant parking space and walk from one end of the mall to the other.

Walk on your vacation and during your lunch hour.

Plan a walking vacation. On your next trip, explore a city by foot. Or make a trip to the mountains, where there's plenty of room to roam.

Walk on your lunch hour. If you're in the city, figure out the longest loop you can take in a nearby park or around several long blocks. If you're in the suburbs, drive to the nearest enclosed mall. You can window shop while you stride briskly around the mall a few times. Some malls even have measured courses marked off for walkers.

Walk to work. Or if that's not possible, park your car as far away as possible and hike the remaining blocks. If you take the train or the bus, just get off a stop earlier – and board one stop later on the way home.

How much exercise is enough? Too little or too much both seem to suppress your immune system. But a good rule of thumb comes from Terry Phillips, Ph.D., director of the Immunogenetics and Immunochemistry Laboratory at George Washington University Medical Center: "There are times when you finish exercising and you get that wonderful sort of euphoric feeling. And then there are other times when you finish and you know it was a real strain." *That's* the difference, he says, between enough and too much, between stimulating the immune system and suppressing it.

Both too little and too much exercise seem to lower your resistance.

Make Sure Your Shots Are up to Date

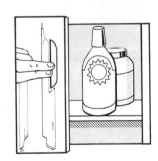

DAY 7

Remember how every fall, just before school started, your mother dragged you to the doctor for booster shots? The school wouldn't let you in unless you were vaccinated against a half dozen different childhood diseases. And you had to produce a note from the doctor to prove it.

Well, listen up, class: Not much has changed, because you *still* need your booster shots. It's the only way to maintain your immunity to several potential killers.

So check your medical records and make sure you're up to date for tetanus and diphtheria. Women of childbearing age should also be immunized against rubella. And older people – plus anyone of any age with heart or respiratory problems – should be immunized against influenza and pneumococcal pneumonia. The pneumonia vaccination is of particular importance, since strains of penicillin-resistant pneumonia have recently developed.

How often do you need these vaccinations? Tetanus and diphtheria vaccinations should be renewed every ten years, doctors advise. But if you've sustained a severe wound, you should get a tetanus booster if your vaccination is more than five years old.

Vaccinations for rubella and pneumococcal pneumonia are necessary only once in your life. But because the flu keeps changing its stripes, you'll need a booster every fall.

We know it hurts. But only for a minute.

Check your medical records to make sure your shots are up to date.

DAY 8

Immune Power Quiz

This immune power quiz will show you how you've done for the first week.

Congratulations! You've finished your first week on our immune power program. Circle the number below that applies and let's see how you've done. (Some factors in the immune power program benefit you more than other factors. For those you receive more points.)

	Never	Sometimes	Always
Do you write in your journal for at least 15 minutes when something upsets you?	1	2	3
Do you practice a relaxation exercise for 20 to 30 minutes once or twice a day?	1	3	5
Did you add foods rich in the B vitamins to your diet?	1	3	5
After you're relaxed, do you visualize a healthy body?	1	2	3
Did you talk about sex with your spouse?	1	2	3
Do you use stairs instead of elevators? Your feet instead of the car?	1	3	5
Have you checked that your shots are up to date?	1	3	5

Total up your score. Then give yourself one of the following ratings: "Immune System Supercharged" if you scored 20 or more points, "Immune System Improved" if you scored from 10 to 19, and "Immune System Sluggish" if you scored anything less than 10.

Count Up Your Selves

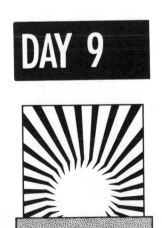

DAY 9

How many "selves" do you have? There's a lot more than just "yourself" wrapped up inside that hundred and whatever-pound body. And discovering who's keeping you company in there can actually increase your resistance to bugs like the flu.

How? Let's find out by taking a look at a study conducted by Patricia Linville, Ph.D., associate professor of psychology at Yale University. Dr. Linville asked 106 students to sit down and think carefully about themselves, then draw up a list of words that described both their negative and positive characteristics.

Students used various adjectives to describe themselves.

One student, for example, described herself as "affectionate," "soft-hearted," "reflective," "impulsive," "competitive," "organized," and "mature." Another student described herself as "lazy," "emotional," "playful," "insecure," "relaxed," and "affectionate."

Dr. Linville transcribed each adjective – there were 33 in all – onto a separate index card. Then, meeting in groups of no more than five people, each student was given the 33 cards that included the self-descriptions, 10 blank cards, and a sheet of legal-size paper with 14 columns.

The students were told to look through the cards, then sort them into groups of characteristics that seemed to belong together. Blank cards were for duplicating any characteristic that belonged in more than one group.

Students who came up with the most "selves" seemed to have the least illness.

When the students were finished, they were asked to record each group of characteristics in one of the columns on the legal-size paper. They did not need to label or name each group, but a look at the students' lists when they were finished revealed that each column actually represented a particular "self" – "me, the child," "me, the friend," "me, the student," "me, the lover," "me, the brother or sister." And, significantly, those with the most "me's" were those who came down with the least number of illnesses.

Focusing on your less stressed "self" can help your immunity.

What's the advantage in knowing how many "me's" there are? You can use that knowledge as a buffer against stress-triggered chemicals that suppress your immune system, explains Dr. Linville. When life is a bowl of cherries for "me, the wife," but little more than the pits for "me, the secretary," you can block the suppression of your immune system simply by focusing on "me, the wife."

It's not just a case of semantics. It's the power of positive feeling. How many "selves" *do* you have?

Take the First Step

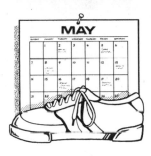

DAY 10

You're already sneaking more walking opportunities into your life, aren't you? Well, now it's time to take a deep breath and make a few more commitments. Commitments to yourself. Commitments to your immune system. Because now that your feet are starting to move, you're going to teach them some new steps.

The first one, if you're over 35 or have any health problems, is to see a doctor. Tell him or her that you want to launch a serious walking program and need to find out if there are any special conditions you should be concerned about. As you become more fit, for example, you may not need as much of a particular medicine that you've been taking.

If you are over 35, talk to your doctor before beginning a serious walking program.

Your second step is one that needs to be taken inside your head: You have to realize that walking is real exercise. You may think you've been doing it all your life, but fitness walking is a skill that you need to develop. If you tried to go out today and walk briskly for an hour, you'd probably end up regretting it for the next week. Your muscles would call out indignantly that

Walking is real exercise, so take precautions.

what you haven't used you have now abused. So we don't want you to hit the ground in full stride. There's too much of a danger that you might quit walking altogether and go back to your old couch potato ways.

ONCE IS NOT ENOUGH

Plan to carry out your walking routine from three to six days a week.

Let's tackle the question of "how often?" first. Regardless of the condition you're in, plan to carry out your walking routine at least three days a week, and not more than six. The reason for the three-day minimum is that any less than that won't give you any conditioning effect. If too many days go by, then you're always starting over and not building strength. And although moderate walks done every day won't hurt you, occasional rest days give your mind and body a rest. If they're built into your plan, you don't have to feel guilty about missing a few days here and there.

Go at your own pace.

Now, how fast and how far should you go? Keep this goal in mind: You want to feel invigorated and relaxed, not fatigued or sore. For some people, that may mean a ½-hour walk covering 1½ miles. For others, it's a 15-minute walk covering ¼ mile. For some of you, it's going to mean walking to the end of the driveway and back.

If you feel winded or out of breath, slow down or stop. Don't be concerned with keeping a steady pace at first. Right now you're just letting your body know you have some new plans for it. And keep in mind that what goes out must come back. Don't walk so far that you can't return without difficulty. If you're not sure how far you can go, keep walking around the block until you have a better idea. That way you'll never be too far from home. Remember, if you're exercising more than you were before, you're getting health benefits, no matter what the speed or distance.

BE CONSCIOUS OF YOUR BODY

While you walk, be aware of your body. Are you hunched over? Are your hands in your pockets or stiff at your sides? Do you tend to lean to the left or the right? Relax and hold your head high. Let your arms swing freely at your sides. Take some deep breaths and relax your shoulders.

Studies have shown that posture can affect people's moods. If you look down, chances are you're feeling down. But by consciously changing how you hold your body, there is a sort of natural biofeedback that says, "Hey, if I'm standing up straight and holding my head high, then I must be feeling good."

There's no right or wrong way for the beginner to walk except by noting what feels comfortable and what doesn't. You'll find that swinging your arms gives you good balance, momentum, and a better overall workout. You may also find that your hands swell due to the blood being forced to your fingertips. It's perfectly natural, but if it bothers you, keep your arms bent at the elbow.

Stand up straight; posture can affect your mood.

ADD AN EXTRA 5 MINUTES

After walking three to five days at whatever pace you've found to be comfortable, try adding an extra 5 minutes to your walk. If that feels okay, that's great. Keep it there for a week or so. If not, drop back to your original distance for another week. Continue adding a few minutes to your walk until you're walking for at least ½ hour, three days a week. When you've reached that goal, start thinking about increasing your speed, but just a tad. At all times let your comfort dictate your speed. You should always be able to carry on a conversation without gasping for breath. Be gentle with yourself, but be consistent.

Periodically increase the time you walk.

Walking at the same time every day can be helpful. But if your schedule is too unpredictable for that or if your personality balks at routine, just promise yourself that sometime that day you'll fit a walk in. Don't do brisk walking before bedtime, though – it'll energize you, not put you to sleep.

KEEP A LOG

Keep a walking log.

Sometimes it's hard to remember just how much you've really walked and how often. That's why it's important to keep a log. Get used to jotting down your walks: how long, how far, how you felt, where you walked. You won't be able to pretend to yourself that you're doing a good job if you're really walking only one day a week. You'll have it down in black and white.

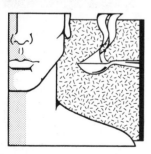

DAY 11   Start a Food Diary

Is there enough zinc roaming your bloodstream to power your antibodies? Are you getting all the B vitamins you need to feed your T-cells?

It's suprisingly easy to think you're getting all the vitamins, minerals, and protein your immune system needs when you're not. The U.S. Department of Agriculture's latest nationwide Continuing Survey of Food Intakes reveals, for example, that American men generally get only 85 percent of the vitamin B₆ they need. Women get only 57 percent of their needed B₆, and little more than half the zinc.

How can you keep tabs on the nutrients that power your immune system? You might want to take a page from a dieter's notebook and start a food diary. Write down everything you eat every day. Then flip to the nutrient tables in a cookbook or other reference just before you go to bed. How much B₆ was in that avocado you had at lunch? How much zinc was in the tomato? *Is* there any zinc in a tomato? Add up the amounts of all the nutrients that are important to your immune system and compare them with the U.S. Recommended Daily Allowances.

How powerful is *your* immune system? Take a look in your diary. You are what you eat. And so is your immune system.

A food diary will tell you whether you're really getting enough vitamins, minerals, and protein.

Read the Comics

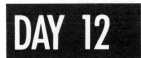

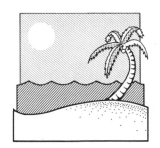

Heard any good jokes lately? How about the one about the drowning man? He went overboard during a squall. A boat came by and offered to pick him up, but the man said, "No, I have faith in the Lord. He'll rescue me any minute." So the boat sailed away.

Pretty soon a helicopter hovered overhead and lowered a sling. But the man waved it away.

"No, thanks. I have faith in the Lord. He'll rescue me any minute." So the helicopter flew away.

Half an hour later, a seaplane landed near the man and offered him a lift. "No thanks," said the man. "I have faith in the Lord, and He'll rescue me *any* minute." So the plane flew away.

Well, not too long after that the man drowned. And when he got to Heaven he demanded an explanation. "Lord! I had such faith! I waited and waited and you never even tried to rescue me!"

The Lord looked at him in amazement. "What do you mean I never tried to rescue you? I sent a boat, a helicopter, and a seaplane!"

Laughter may be good for your immune system.

Got a chuckle out of that one, did you? Good. Because whether it's a chuckle from a comic strip, a delighted grin at a friend's frantic antics, or a belly laugh from a Bill Cosby video, laughter – believe it or not – is good for your immune system.

When you're under pressure, laughter may boost your immune function.

Scientists are not quite at the stage where they will say a laugh a day will keep the doctor away. But they do know that if you're sitting in an office under pressure and you get upset about it, your immune function will go down. Approach the situation with humor, and your immune function will go up.

How do they know? They know because they measured the concentration of antibodies in a group of ten students who were watching videotapes – one funny (*Richard Pryor Live*) and one boring (an educational tape on anxiety). The results? The students' antibody levels remained the same both before and after viewing the educational tape. But they shot *up* after watching Richard Pryor.

Why did the lobster blush? 'Cause he saw the salad dressing.

Laughter may increase your production of lymphocytes.

Oops! Gotcha again, didn't we? Good. Your laughter may have just blocked the shot of an immunosuppressive chemical directed at your

T-cells. Or it may have increased your production of lymphocyte warriors. Maybe it did both.

A joint study by a psychiatrist at Stanford University and an immunologist at Loma Linda University Medical Center revealed that either is possible. William Fry, M.D., of Stanford, and Lee Berk, of Loma Linda, rounded up ten healthy students and divided them into two groups.

The first group watched a 60-minute videotape of the comedian Gallagher, while the second group twiddled their thumbs. Blood samples were taken from each student before, during, and after the video and thumb-twiddling, then analyzed for 30 or 40 different substances that would tell the investigators how laughter affected the students' immune systems – if it did at all.

Blood samples were taken from students who watched videotapes of comedies.

It did. When Berk compared the samples from the two groups in his lab, he found that laughter had increased the production of lymphocyte warriors by 39 percent and decreased by 46 percent the amount of cortisol – a stress hormone produced by the body that suppresses major players in the immune system.

Laughter, the researchers concluded, had cut the effects of everyday stress on the students' immune systems almost in half. And it had turbocharged the process by which their bodies produce fresh troops.

Laughter cut the effects of everyday stress almost in half.

So what's the easiest way to keep your immune system in stitches? "Everybody has a somewhat different sense of humor," says Dr. Fry, who admits that he and his colleagues keep *their* immune systems alert by playing practical jokes.

The best way to use laughter to boost immune function is to take a humor inventory. "Some people like Laurel and Hardy, some like the Three Stooges," he says. "Get a reading on your sense of humor and find out what's funny to you. Then collect a humor library: books, cartoons, tapes, films, audios, objects, anything.

Find out what's funny to you and collect a humor library.

"I have one particular object that I like to play with," chuckles the scientist. "You know how a balloon shoots around the room when you let it go? Well, this is like a balloon with a gyroscope. It has propellers, and it shoots up in the air and then around the *world*." He laughs. "You should see it," he says – and gives his immune system another charge of chuckles.

"Have you ever been to a clown funeral?" asked comedian Steve Wright. "Everybody goes in the same car!"

DAY 13

Put Yourself on a Sleep Schedule

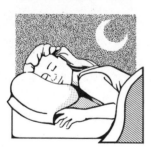

You need a good night's sleep to give your immune system a chance to regenerate itself.

In the black reaches of the outer galaxy, astronauts won't have a rising or a setting sun to tell them when it's time to hit the deck or hit the hay. So scientists plan to put them on a sleep schedule – complete with snooze alarms and wake-up calls – as compatible as possible with their natural biorhythms.

Fortunately, you don't have to wait for intergalactic travel before you get a good night's sleep. Just borrow the rhythm method from our space program. Figure out what your natural sleep schedule is, scientists say, then program your body to follow it by going to bed at the same time every night and getting up at the same time every morning. Creatures of habit apparently get a good night's sleep. And that's important if you want to give your immune system a chance to regenerate itself.

But don't fall into the trap of thinking that unless you get 8 hours of shut-eye every night your biorhythms will take a turn for the worse. True, the average amount of sleep for adults is 7 to 8 hours a night. But the range of sleep requirements for individuals is vast – from about 6 to 9 hours for 90 percent of the population. A few people may need only 5 hours of sleep. Others may need as much as 10.

Unfortunately, confusion about real sleep requirements has forced some people into a kind of false insomnia: You think you must get 8 hours of sleep each night, yet your body really needs only 6, so you fret about taking so long to fall asleep or waking up so early.

"Each person has a genetically determined sleep requirement," explains Merrill M. Mitler, Ph.D., a sleep expert at the University of California, San Diego. "As far as we know, this need doesn't change during adulthood and can't be reduced by 'practice.' The notion that the elderly need less sleep is probably based on the fact that they often get less sleep because of medical problems."

If you don't know what your sleep requirement is, try this: For one month, get the same amount of sleep each night, retiring and rising at precisely the same time. Assess how you feel on this schedule. Then for two weeks, get 30 minutes more or less sleep per night and see if you feel better or worse during the day. Keep up this kind of trial and error until you pin down your RSA – your Recommended Snooze Allowance.

Then, once you do, put yourself on a sleep schedule: down at the same time every night, up at the same time every morning.

And, yes, even on weekends.

The range of sleep requirements for individuals is vast.

Use trial and error to determine your RSA—your Recommended Snooze Allowance.

DAY 14

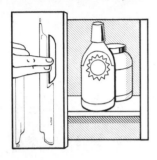

Overexposure to sunlight suppresses the immune system.

Sunscreens prevent the immunosuppressive effects of sunlight.

Use a waterproof sunscreen with the highest SPF you can find.

Buy Yourself a Sunscreen

Around the middle of the 20th century, bronze skin became a badge of wealth – a sign that you had the money and time to frolic in the sun. But in this, the latter part of the 20th century, a deep tan has become the sign of doubtful intelligence.

Research has proven that the short-term effect of overexposure to sunlight is a suppressed immune system that can leave you open to all sorts of microscopic invaders. And the long-term effect is skin cancer.

Fortunately, an ounce of prevention is not only worth a pound of cure, it also comes in a variety of lotions, gels, oils, and mousses that you rub on, spray on, smooth on and slather over your body. It comes in the form of sunscreens.

"Sunscreens prevent the immunosuppressive effects of sunlight," says Warwick Morison, M.D., associate professor of dermatology at Johns Hopkins University. Rather than acting like a physical filter or screen – as their name implies – they actually work chemically by binding to the skin and providing a barrier against the damaging part of sunlight.

How much should you use? Actually, "We really don't have a good handle on how much to use," says Dr. Morison. "It depends on the color of your skin, how you tan, and how much exposure you get."

The best way to protect yourself is to use a waterproof sunscreen with the highest SPF (sun protection factor) number you can find. And don't count on the moisturizers, tints, and make-ups to guard you. They may protect your skin from wrinkles, says Dr. Morison, but they won't keep your immune system on the job.

If you're dark, tan easily, and don't go out in the sun a lot, he adds, you need a sunscreen only when you're ready to hit the beach. If you're fair and in the sun a lot, using a sunscreen on a daily basis during the summer isn't a bad idea.

Immune Power Quiz DAY 15

Congratulations! You've finished your second week on our immune power program. Circle the number below that applies and let's see how you've done.

	Never	Sometimes	Always
Do you write in your journal for at least 15 minutes when something upsets you?	1	2	3
Do you practice a relaxation exercise for 20 to 30 minutes once or twice a day?	1	3	5
Do you eat foods rich in the B vitamins?	1	3	5
After you're relaxed, do you visualize a healthy body?	1	2	3
Did you count up your "selves"?	1	2	3
Do you walk at least three times a week?	1	3	5
Did you start a food diary?	1	3	5

(continued)

	Never	Sometimes	Always
Did you take a humor inventory?	1	2	3
Are you getting up and going to bed at the same time every day?	1	3	5
Do you use a sunscreen?	1	3	5

Total up your score. Then give yourself one of the following ratings: "Immune System Supercharged" if you scored 30 or more points, "Immune System Improved" if you scored from 14 to 29, and "Immune System Sluggish" if you scored anything less than 14.

DAY 16

Ban Smoking from Your Environment

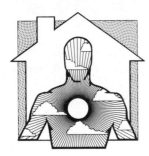

If a smoker lights up, passive-aggressive behavior is not the way to respond.

Smoking is no longer a social issue arbitrated by Miss Manners. It reduces the effectiveness of your immune system whether you're the smoker or the innocent bystander.

How can we convince the smokers among us of our inalienable right to smoke-free air? By speaking up. The right way.

Let's say you're sitting in a restaurant and a smoker lights up nearby. Your typical response – coughing, waving your hands, maybe grumbling – is called passive-aggressive behavior. And it's the worst possible course, says psychologist Barry Lubetkin, Ph.D., director of the Institute for Behavior Therapy in New York City.

"People have the most resistance to change when others aren't completely frank with them. If someone waves away the smoke but doesn't say anything to the smoker, it gives the smoker a chance to disengage himself from responsibility for his act," he says.

In fact, he says, passive-aggressive behavior often angers the smoker more than a request. Why? "Everybody has had the experience, often as children, of people making comments or gestures about them behind their backs. We tend to respond with fury. But if you confront the smoker politely, he must take responsibility for what he's doing. And if you can provide him with an alternative that saves face, it generally works."

It is better to confront the smoker politely.

Dr. Lubetkin suggests that you try one of these lines:

- "I would appreciate it if you blew your smoke in another direction."
- "I understand that you want to continue smoking and that's fine. But could you hold your cigarette in your other hand?"
- "We'll be leaving in 10 minutes. If you can hold off smoking until then, we'd appreciate it."

If these don't work, escalate your request, says Dr. Lubetkin:

If necessary, escalate to a firmer request.

- "Would you mind putting out your cigarette? This is a no-smoking area."
- "Excuse me, I'm allergic to cigarette smoke (or, I have trouble breathing cigarette smoke) and I must ask you to put out your cigarette."

Virtually all smokers will comply with these last two lines, says Dr. Lubetkin. If they don't, escalate a little more by asking your waiter or waitress to make the request.

In the rare instance where all requests fail, ask to be moved to another table. Then when you finish your meal, write a note on your check to the manager. Tell him what happened. And tell him that you won't be back until the air has been cleared.

Let restaurant managers know if you have a problem with cigarette smoke.

DAY 17

Act Like a "Cockeyed Optimist"

You may not look like Sally Sunshine, but climbing into the pink-and-white gingham pinafore of her optimism may help your immune system block some nasty shots from a stressful world.

How? Scientists really aren't sure. What they are sure of is that people who are optimistic get sick far less often than the rest of us Dour Donnas.

That doesn't mean you have to force yourself into the cheery emotional state of Mitzi Gaynor, the "cockeyed optimist" in *South Pacific*. But if you want a zipped-up immune system, it does mean that you should at least study the way Gaynor's character handled her problems. Then copy some of her techniques.

How *does* an optimist handle problems? The natural inclination of an optimist is to meet any problem head on, reveals Michael Scheier, Ph.D., a researcher at Carnegie-Mellon University. She doesn't waste time denying that a problem exists or worrying about its implications. Instead she defines it, focuses on it, deals with it, and makes a deliberate attempt to dwell on the good things in any resulting situation.

She also accepts things she cannot change, Dr. Scheier says. Ultimately a pragmatist, the optimist figures there's no sense in getting bent out of shape about something she can't do anything about.

Say you're an optimist and your gynecologist tells you that your latest Pap smear indicates

Optimism gives your immune system some zip.

Optimists meet problems head on.

a cancerous condition. Your hands and feet turn to ice. Your hearing seems to diminish. Your doctor seems far away. But a few seconds later your mind manages to get around the edges of its terror and ask the necessary questions: What can I do about it? How long will the treatment take? When will I get back to work?

Once your questions are answered, your decisions made, your plans in gear, you buy a bunch of books for your convalescence and reschedule all your appointments. You don't cancel them, of course. Why should you? You'll deal with the cancer, get a good rest, and catch up with all those books that you've been too busy to read.

The optimist even faces up to cancer.

Your optimist's mind is already on the future. And, since your immune system is gearing up to make it happen, chances are your body will be there, too.

Rethink Veggies DAY 18

Eat a carrot. Munch on broccoli. Wrap your tongue around a wad of grape leaves. You may begin to feel like Bugs Bunny, but if you want a strong immune system, you're going to have to eat your veggies.

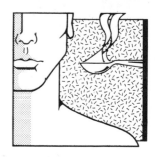

Think yellow, orange, and green.

You have to because your body takes vegetables and breaks them down into chemical components that help immune system cells grow up and turn into warriors.

What kinds of vegetables should you be eating? Those that are yellow or orange in color are especially good bets, and so are leafy greens. They contain high amounts of beta-carotene, a substance your body converts to vitamin A. And vitamin A is necessary for the production and maturation of various immune system fighters.

Fortunately, it's easy to load up on vitamin A. A single raw carrot, for example, provides about 20,000 international units (IU) of vitamin A. The U.S. Recommended Daily Allowance for vitamin A is only 5,000 IU. So three bites of carrot and your immune warriors should be ready to hit the warpath.

Sweet potatoes and greens are packed with nutrients.

Another good immune power veggie is a baked sweet potato. Not only does it provide about 25,000 IU of vitamin A, it also has small amounts of vitamin C, calcium, copper, iron, and magnesium. You can drop it, as is, on your dinner plate or turn it into some scrumptious sweet potato bread.

If you're not into sweet potatoes, you might add a cup of greens – such as collard or turnip – to your plate instead. And before you turn up your nose, you should know that a cup of cooked turnip greens translates into 7,918 IU of vitamin A and a kiss each of vitamin C, calcium, iron, magnesium, and copper. A cup of raw turnip greens has slightly less value, but thrown together with carrots into what you might call a "southern salad," the combination can be immune-power dynamite.

DAY 19

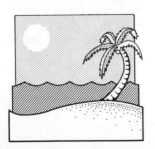

Learn How to Play

Play. How many of us remember how to play jacks? Throw a boomerang? Draw a hopscotch? Yet scientists tell us that childhood games may improve the function of our adult immune systems simply by throwing stress to the mat. So pick a childhood game that is totally fun and totally without merit in the adult world and go for it.

Need some help? Red light/green light is, according to game pro Tommy Childers, age 6, a game that requires quick feet, quick responses, and a stout pair of lungs. One person pretends to be a traffic light and stands 20 feet or so from the rest of the children who are, presumably, the cars. The traffic light yells, "Green light!" and the children run as fast as they can toward the traffic light. The traffic light yells, "Red light!" and the children screech to a halt. Anyone who doesn't stop is sent back to the parking lot.

No matter how short the traffic light makes the time between his call of "Red light!" and "Green light!" eventually one of the children will come close enough to touch – or, in some versions, run past – the traffic light. Whoever does, of course, is the next traffic light, able to order his playmates around with impunity.

Think it's a little – ah – simplistic? Good. Then maybe it's exactly what you need.

Childhood games, like red light/green light, may improve the function of our adult immune systems.

Lean into Fitness

DAY 20

Now that your feet have found their walking rhythm, let's see if they're ready for the next step in immune system fitness. Begin with a mental image. Picture yourself in a tunnel inside an Egyptian pyramid. You've just discovered an ancient cart loaded with gold jewelry and precious stones.

If you can manage to get that cart outside, its cargo is yours to keep. The only problem is

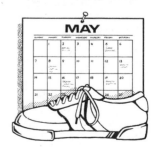

that the wheels on the cart have grown fragile with the rust of centuries. If you push it too hard, those ancient wheels are just liable to shatter under the strain, and you'll never get your treasure. So you don't push at all. What you do is *lean*. You lean against that cart until it begins to move, ever so slowly. And you keep leaning. You don't get impatient and start shoving, no matter how slowly the cart moves, because time doesn't really matter. Only progress matters. If you get tired, you rest. Then you carry on, leaning, getting your precious cargo closer to the end of the tunnel.

Lean into an advanced walking program; don't push it.

That's how you go after advanced fitness walking. You *lean* into it. You don't push. You take your time.

Now with that image ever in mind, get an inexpensive digital sports watch – you can find one for under $15 – lace up your sneaks, and find a walking course that's about 1 mile long or that takes you about 15 to 20 minutes to cover at your usual walking speed. The exact distance isn't important – just be sure to make note of start and stop landmarks at both ends.

Ideally, the course you choose will be a segment of the route you're already walking as part of your regular fitness routine – or a convenient detour from it. The terrain should be smooth and fairly flat, and your route must be free from traffic interruptions.

Begin your program by recording your time at your *usual* pace.

All set? The first time you try advanced fitness walking, just include your special fitness course as part of your usual walk. When you reach the start point, start the stopwatch. Continue walking at your *usual speed* to the end of the course, then freeze your time. Make a note of it in the walking log you started on Day 10. This is your base time for the course. And next week you're going to top it.

Pick the Right Vitamin Supplement

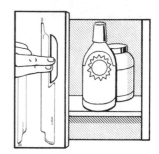

DAY 21

How many cups of kale can you eat in a day? No, it's not the beginning of another joke. It's the beginning of understanding. Of understanding just how much food it takes to power your body's immune system.

Consider the U.S. Recommended Daily Allowance for magnesium. It's 400 milligrams. Yet a cup of kale – which is loaded with other immune system nutrients such as vitamin A – has only 23 milligrams. So what are you going to do? Eat 17 cups of cooked kale?

You could, of course, choose another vegetable. One higher in magnesium. Well, a cup of cooked spinach has 158 milligrams of magnesium. That's getting closer. But it would still take 2½ cups of the warm, wet stuff to meet your body's basic requirements. And, even if you love spinach, 2½ cups is a bit much.

It seems to come down to one basic choice: either spend most of your day grazing in the kitchen and feeling like you're the little piggy being fattened for market, or get the most nutrients you can from three squares a day and take a vitamin supplement to cover anything you may have missed.

You may want to take a vitamin supplement to cover nutrients you may have missed.

Which supplement is right for you? "As long as you're eating a reasonable diet, one of those standard daily multivitamins is sufficient"

A standard multivitamin is probably sufficient.

to keep your immune system at maximum efficiency, says Dr. Phillips from George Washington University Medical Center.

DAY 22   Immune Power Quiz

Congratulations! You've finished your third week on our immune power program. Circle the number below that applies and let's see how you've done.

	Never	Sometimes	Always
Do you write in your journal for at least 15 minutes when something upsets you?	1	2	3
Do you practice a relaxation exercise for 20 to 30 minutes once or twice a day?	1	3	5
Do you eat foods rich in the B vitamins?	1	3	5
After you're relaxed, do you visualize a healthy body?	1	2	3
Do you concentrate on your positive "selves"?	1	3	5
Do you walk at least three times a week?	1	3	5
Do you keep a food diary?	1	3	5
Are you building a humor "library"?	1	2	3

	Never	**Sometimes**	**Always**
Are you getting up and going to bed at the same time every day?	1	3	5
Do you use a sunscreen?	1	3	5
Have you banned cigarette smoke from your environment?	1	3	5
Do you act like an optimist, even when you feel like a grump?	1	2	3
Did you add foods rich in vitamin A to your diet?	1	3	5
Did you play a childhood game?	1	2	3
Did you add the 1-mile course to your walk?	1	3	5
Did you buy a multivitamin supplement?	1	3	5

Total up your score. Then give yourself one of the following ratings: "Immune System Supercharged" if you scored 60 or more points, "Immune System Improved" if you scored from 25 to 59, and "Immune System Sluggish" if you scored anything less than 25.

Get Rid of Antisleep Habits

DAY 23

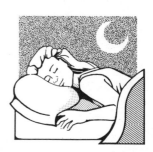

Now that you've been on a sleep schedule for the past 10 days, let's take a look at how you're doing.

How are you doing on your sleep schedule?

Are you nodding off right after your head touches the pillow? Are you refreshed by the time you've spent in bed? If you answered yes, great. But don't feel bad if you're tossing and turning so much that you're beginning to feel like a rumpled blanket. You're not alone.

Many Americans suffer from insomnia.

At any given time, 120 million Americans may suffer from so-called transient insomnia, the kind that lasts less than three weeks and is caused by short-term, simple stress. Then there are an additional 20 million victims who endure chronic insomnia: long-term poor sleep caused by physical or behavioral problems.

But whether you call them transient or chronic, all these insomniacs take too long to fall asleep (generally 30 minutes or more), have trouble staying asleep (awaken too many times or too early), or experience sleep that's too light.

The causes are many, but the problem is more manageable than many people think.

What causes these problems? The most common causes of insomnia have more to do with your own head than with dripping faucets or noisy neighbors. Depression, anxiety, stress, tension, psychoses – these force people to sleep-disorder centers in droves.

The problems are also frequently more manageable than many people think. Severe depression and other serious psychological problems require and often respond to professional help. Mild stress and anxiety usually ease up with relaxation techniques, regular exercise, or biofeedback. And certain behavioral sleep-stoppers disappear with regular doses of behavioral countermeasures.

A stressful day, for example, makes it tough for you to fall asleep. So you try harder. And the harder you try, the more uptight you get – becoming more wide-eyed by the hour. So you stop trying. And as you switch on the TV to watch the 4:00 A.M. farm news, you doze off.

The moral? You can't force sleep. So do the opposite, say sleep experts. When you can't drift off, get out of bed and get your mind off sleep. Read, watch TV, knit. And when you finally feel sleepy, return to bed. The next day, rise at your standard time (no matter how late you stayed up) and avoid daytime naps unless they're part of your usual routine. Otherwise you may end up reversing your body's sleep/wake schedule, sleeping in and retiring later and later.

Then there's this behavioral mixup: Your darkened bedroom, your comfy pillow, your bedtime ritual of brushing your teeth or reading a book don't trigger sleep as they do in many people – instead they stir you up, actually keep you from sleeping. But when you're on the sofa, or when you skip your usual bedtime routine – while traveling, for instance – you can doze off in nothing flat. What's wrong?

Psychologists call it maladaptive conditioning. If your bedroom is a pressure cooker where the frustrations of insomnia or daily stress heat up, you can begin to associate it with wakefulness rather than rest. Often you can get into this odd predicament by doing everything in the world in bed except sleeping – talking on the phone, working, writing letters, paying bills, worrying about tomorrow, eating, watching TV – or simply lying in bed fretting about your lack of sleep.

MAKE NEW CONNECTIONS

You get out of this mess by breaking the sleep-stopping connections and forming better ones. You start by using your bed *only* for sleeping and sex and by going to bed only when you're really sleepy. If you hop into bed and then start to feel restless, use the nonforced sleep technique mentioned above, even if it means getting out of bed a dozen times.

You can't force sleep.

Maybe you associate your bedroom with wakefulness rather than rest.

Try using your bed *only* for sleeping and sex.

During the first night of this new conditioning, you probably won't sleep much. But any loss of shut-eye will help you sleep better the next night. By the third night, you'll probably drop off to dreamland on the first or second try. Then you can resume the natural rhythms of your sleep schedule. And not feel like a rumpled blanket.

DAY 24

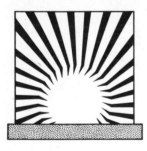

Learning the "Relaxation Response" can benefit your immune system.

Regenerate Your Spirit

What do a Tibetan monk, a Philadelphia Quaker, and a Methodist minister have in common? The ability to enter a deeply relaxed state of consciousness that – in their own individual terms – alters their state of being. And while each seeker's consciousness is being altered by prayer or meditation, so are naturally produced body chemicals that can affect the immune system.

How can you manipulate these chemicals to achieve the immune equivalent of nirvana? Herbert Benson, M.D., an associate professor of medicine at Harvard Medical School, has studied and written extensively on what he has dubbed the "Relaxation Response" and the "Faith Factor." And in his book *Your Maximum Mind,* he suggests that you focus your mind on a word or short phrase that's firmly rooted in your spiritual belief system – "shalom" if you're Jewish, for example, or "praise the Lord" if you're a Christian or, for the nonreligious, a word such as "peace."

Then twice a day, for 10 minutes at a time, sit down in a comfortable position, close your eyes, and relax your muscles. Breathe slowly, and as you exhale, silently repeat your focus word or phrase. Don't worry if your mind is distracted or wanders away toward another thought. Even another world. Gently bring it back to your focus word.

It won't be long before your immune system is a believer.

Practice relaxation twice a day, 10 minutes at a time.

Visit the Fish Market

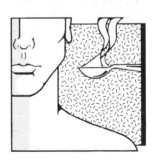

DAY 25

Eat fish to make sure you're getting enough zinc and protein.

Two things your immune system simply cannot live without are zinc and protein. Yet most women in the United States get barely half of the 15 milligrams of zinc their bodies need every day. And anyone who goes on a diet probably isn't getting enough protein to fuel their immune systems either.

How can you make sure your natural killer cells have enough zinc and protein to fight off an invader? The answer may be a visit to your local fish market. One-third cup of raw eastern oysters or breaded, microwavable oysters gives you about 75 milligrams of zinc.

Shellfish and other seafood are also a good source of protein. Depending on your weight, you may need 40 to 60 grams or more of protein a day. And if you're pregnant, nursing, stressed out, or infected, you need even more – ask your doctor for a recommendation.

But grams of protein don't mean much to most of us. So the American Heart Association recommends that you simply remember to get two servings of meat, poultry, seafood, nuts, dried beans, peas, or eggs every day. That's the equivalent of one chicken breast, a cup of flaked fish, or four thin slices of lean roast beef.

Anyone for poached salmon?

Eat two servings of meat, poultry, seafood, nuts, dried beans, peas, or eggs every day.

DAY 26 Ditch Your Pesticides

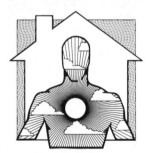

Pesticides are designed to overwhelm the defense systems of bugs. But they can also damage yours. Laboratory studies indicate that pesticides can lower the numbers of T-cells that turn your immune system on and off, slow down your macrophages, and disarm the natural killers you depend on to root out bacteria, viruses, and tumors.

Given the effects of pesticides, the pests begin to look good.

What can you do besides practice interspe-cies toleration? How can you do unto others without getting it done unto you?

Natural alternatives may be the answer. Use flyswatters in the living room, ant traps under the bed, boric acid behind the hot-water tank, Japanese beetle traps on the lawn, burlap cum-berbunds around the trees, and sprays of soapy water in the garden. Pouring boiling water on the nests of ants and sprinkling diatoma-ceous earth around the house perimeter will also reduce the invasion of things that creep and crawl.

Natural alternatives may prevent pesticide damage.

You can even use a natural alternative to keep your cat pest-free. In a study at the Ohio State University Department of Entomology, researchers found that linalool, a colorless, woodsy-smelling liquid found in citrus peel oil, killed every adult flea on cats that had been dipped in a 1-percent solution. Nylon carpet squares – which were deliberately infested with eggs, larvae, and adult fleas in the lab – were sprayed with a 5 percent solution. It could have been napalm as far as the fleas were concerned. Not one flea survived. And even though this naturally occurring substance is a potent pest-fighter, its toxicity to humans appears low.

Linalool is a natural alterna-tive to keep your cat pest-free.

Your most effective weapons in the war against creepy, crawly things, however, are still your hands and your head. Your hands can pick any objectionable critters off a plant or a base-board (sneak around with a flashlight to sur-prise the nocturnal ones, garden experts suggest), and your head can figure out how to outfox them. If the codling moth is decimating your apple trees, for example, hang up a block of suet. The suet will invite every woodpecker within flying distance for dinner. Guess what they like for dessert?

Pick creepy, crawly things off by hand and figure out how to outfox them.

DAY 27

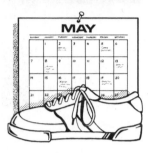

Speed Up Your Immune System

The next time you're ready for a walk, go back to the course you established on Day 20 of our program. But this time, warm up first. Walk at a normal, easy pace for about 15 minutes, take several deep breaths along the way, flap your arms around, rotate your shoulders, swivel your hips. That sort of thing.

Begin your walking session after warming up.

Having warmed up, go back to your start point, hit the button on your stopwatch and begin your walking again. For the first 5 minutes, proceed at the same speed you did the first time you walked the course. At the 5-minute mark, though, pick up your speed. Don't do that by taking longer strides. Longer strides only strain your muscles. Just move your legs faster. A *little* faster. Don't pump your arms or do anything other than take faster strides. After about 4 or 5 minutes, return to your normal pace and continue to the end of your course. Stop your watch.

Check how you feel before you check your stopwatch.

Don't check your time yet. Check yourself. Does anything ache? Are you winded? Do you feel strange? If you feel anything other than great, you're not ready for advanced fitness walking. Carry on with your usual walking, and try again in a month. If you feel really bad, see a physician. Probably, though, you'll feel just fine.

Now check that time on your stopwatch. Ideally, you've shaved 10 or 15 seconds from your time. If your time is the same as it was last

week, don't worry. Try again tomorrow or the
next day. If you can take those 10 or 15 seconds
off your time then, you're really on your way to
fitness.

Get a Lymphocyte Check

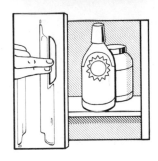

DAY 28

Your immune system knows when something's about to go bad. Even if the rest of you
hasn't a clue and your latest checkup says you're
okay, your immune system can apparently detect
any life-threatening assault at the cellular level.

"In one study we did, we found that the
number of lymphocytes declined three years
before a patient died," says William H. Adler,
M.D., chief of clinical immunology at the National
Institute on Aging. And it didn't matter whether
patients died from a heart attack, pneumonia,
cancer, or influenza. Their lymphocytes started
signaling an alarm three years in advance.

How do you detect a lymphocyte drop?
"Look at the lab slip next time your doctor
orders a blood test," Dr. Adler suggests. Multiply
the number marked "percent of lymphocytes"
by the number marked "white count." That gives
you the number of lymphocytes per milliliter of
blood. Then keep a record of each test so you
can detect any change, or ask your doctor to
do it.

**Your lymphocyte count can
serve as an early warning
system.**

A drop in count is what you want to watch for.

But don't expect a big change. The actual number of lymphocytes isn't what's important – it's the drop. "The changes in our studies weren't something that a doctor would raise his eyebrows at," says Dr. Adler. "They were gradual. Within normal limits."

Rather than using the test as a predictor of death, says Dr. Adler, you should use it as an indicator of danger. You can use it as a kind of early warning system and go hunting for the problem. Ask your doctor to order a computerized axial tomography (CAT) scan or a positron emission tomography (PET) scan and take a closer look. Maybe he can figure out what's wrong. Maybe, together, you can fix it.

DAY 29

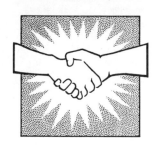

Make the World a Better Place

Trusting and caring for other people may have a powerful effect on the immune system.

When Boston University's David McClelland, Ph.D., showed films of Mother Teresa in action to college students, a strange thing happened. He discovered that just *watching* people do good deeds resulted in higher levels of antibody warriors in some of the students. And it didn't matter whether the students admired Mother Teresa or not, says Dr. McClelland. Even if they thought she was misguided, their immune systems treated her like a saint.

How can *you* reap the immune system benefits of caring? Just look around. There are always people in need, people to whom a child's outgrown jeans or a woman's I-no-longer-need-it maternity dress are a blessing. There are always soup kitchens that can use an extra bag of groceries and hospitals that can use an extra pair of hands.

You can read for the blind, walk for the old, cook for the ill. Helping them could help your immune system.

Your immune system will reap the benefits of caring.

Immune Power Final Exam

DAY 30

Way to go! You've finished 30 days on our immune power program. Circle the number below that applies and let's see how you've done.

	Never	Sometimes	Always
Do you write in your journal for at least 15 minutes when something upsets you?	1	2	3
Do you practice a relaxation exercise for 20 to 30 minutes once or twice a day?	1	3	5
Do you eat foods rich in the B vitamins?	1	3	5
After you're relaxed, do you visualize a healthy body?	1	2	3

(continued)

	Never	Sometimes	Always
Do you concentrate on your positive "selves"?	1	3	5
Do you walk at least three times a week?	1	3	5
Do you keep a food diary?	1	3	5
Are you building a humor "library"?	1	2	3
Are you getting up and going to bed at the same time every day?	1	3	5
Do you use a sunscreen?	1	3	5
Have you maintained a smoke-free environment?	1	3	5
Do you act like an optimist, even when you feel like a grump?	1	2	3
Do you eat foods rich in vitamin A?	1	3	5
Do you play childhood games?	1	2	3
Do you take a multivitamin?	1	3	5
Have you tried to use the "Faith Factor"?	1	2	3
Do you visit the fish market?	1	3	5
Did you ditch your pesticides?	1	3	5
Did you subtract 15 seconds from your walking program?	1	3	5
Do you know how many lymphocytes you have on the job?	1	3	5
Do you do a good deed every day?	1	2	3

Total up your score. Then give yourself one of the following ratings: "Immune System Supercharged" if you scored 80 or more points, "Immune System Improved" if you scored from 50 to 80, and "Immune System Sluggish" if you scored anything less than 50.

INDEX

Rodale Press, Inc., publishes PREVENTION, America's leading health magazine.
For information on how to order your subscription,
write to PREVENTION, Emmaus, PA 18098.